I0791665

LIVING LONGER AND REVERSING AGING

A Prescription for a Healthier and Longer Life

Jairo A. Puentes, M.D.

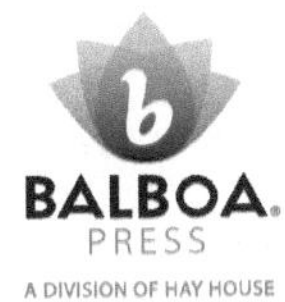

BALBOA.
PRESS

A DIVISION OF HAY HOUSE

This book is a work of non-fiction. Unless otherwise noted, the author and the publisher make no explicit guarantees as to the accuracy of the information contained in this book and in some cases, names of people and places have been altered to protect their privacy.

The information, ideas, and suggestions in this book are not intended as a substitute for professional medical advice. Before following any suggestions contained in this book, you should consult your personal physician. Neither the author nor the publisher shall be liable or responsible for any loss or damage allegedly arising as a consequence of your use or application of any information or suggestions in this book.

Balboa Press books may be ordered through booksellers or by contacting:

Balboa Press
A Division of Hay House
1663 Liberty Drive
Bloomington, IN 47403
www.balboapress.com
1 (877) 407-4847

Because of the dynamic nature of the Internet, any web addresses or links contained in this book may have changed since publication and may no longer be valid. The views expressed in this work are solely those of the author and do not necessarily reflect the views of the publisher, and the publisher hereby disclaims any responsibility for them.

The author of this book does not dispense medical advice or prescribe the use of any technique as a form of treatment for physical, emotional, or medical problems without the advice of a physician, either directly or indirectly. The intent of the author is only to offer information of a general nature to help you in your quest for emotional and spiritual well-being. In the event you use any of the information in this book for yourself, which is your constitutional right, the author and the publisher assume no responsibility for your actions.

Print information available on the last page.

ISBN: 978-1-9822-1446-3 (sc)
ISBN: 978-1-9822-1448-7 (hc)
ISBN: 978-1-9822-1447-0 (e)

Library of Congress Control Number: 2018912602

Balboa Press rev. date: 10/27/2018

*To my beautiful wife, Clara, my coauthor and wonderful companion.
You have been my inspiration from the time I met you and have
given me such valuable assistance in writing this book.
I hope the love and happiness we have enjoyed together may inspire others reading
this book to find the same as they travel with us on this beautiful planet.*

CONTENTS

ACKNOWLEDGMENTS

Writing a book is a work of love. Writing a nonfiction book is not an easy task. It requires reading hundreds of books, magazines, and newspapers and performing just as many searches in the internet. It also requires reviews by friends and colleagues for feedback. I was fortunate my wife loves reading books. She particularly likes nutritional and self-help books. Her contribution has been immense. She reads a new book every week and selects areas or passages of special interest for me to review. This prescreening saved me lots of time. I felt it was fair to add her name as a coauthor, since her advice and contribution has been immense.

The idea for this book also came from my wife's good looks. Most of our friends are amazed about her health, beauty, and youth. She seems to be aging at a very slow pace and her chronological age doesn't match her biological or psychological age. She looks decades younger. Well, may be something of what she does is helping me as well, since I look younger too.

I have to recognize many people in my life for helping me to be where I am now—full of life, energy, and wisdom. Besides my wife, who is the love of my life, I must acknowledge my parents, who gave me a great education that allowed me to become a medical doctor. My mother in particularly deserves special recognition. She gave me a great deal of love to build my confidence and character, which to this date has been the greatest gift a parent can give to a child.

I was also surrounded by aunts and uncles who were teachers who helped me to advance in knowledge and compassion.

I am grateful to my high school teachers at the De La Salle Brothers school I attended, who gave me such a great education and Christian values.

From them, I learned the value of prayer, love, and compassion for the poor and those suffering because of poverty or illness. They recognized my dedication by giving me the highest honor upon graduation from high school. I was the valedictorian and received many accolades. This preparation they gave me was invaluable to pass the admission process and exam to get into medical school, and to this date, their influence is reflected in my work.

I had numerous professors who enlightened me and gave me meaningful advice. To all of them, I am very grateful. I also was privileged to have my specialty training at the University of Pennsylvania, where I had great teachers. They were outstanding clinicians who had a lot of influence in my future professional development. I will always be grateful to my boss, William Erdman, MD, for accepting me at Penn. I am grateful to one of my mentors and a tremendous supporter, Professor Eleanor Bendler, MD, from whom I learned so much to become a dedicated clinician searching for the truth. She gave me great letters of recommendation that eventually had an incredible impact in my professional life. Because of her recommendations, I was accepted to become a member of the faculty of Baylor College of Medicine, where I taught medicine for fourteen years.

I am grateful to my former boss and director at Baylor College of Medicine, Professor Lewis Levitt, MD, for his confidence in me and his guidance.

I am also grateful to my friends in Houston, partners in the development of nutritional and cardiac rehabilitation programs at the Travis Medical Center in Houston. Dr. Denton Cooley, MD, the renowned cardiovascular surgeon, took me under his wing and allowed me to create and develop exercise and nutritional programs for cardiac patients and elite athletes at the medical center in Houston. Dr. Stanley Dudrick, MD, counseled and mentored me in the use of hyperalimentation and research in nutrition of pre and postsurgical patients.

Without all these mentors and opportunities, it would have been difficult for me to learn so much about nutrition, exercise, and preventive care. My experience as an exercise expert and teacher at Baylor gave me opportunity to treat patients with severe disabilities and chronic pain. This experience has been invaluable. After fourteen years of teaching, I was able to apply all this knowledge and experience to open two outpatient clinics and build a rehabilitation hospital in Corpus Christi. This book reflects all these years of experience in an effort to help people to live a better and healthier life and reverse many changes related to the aging process.

I also want to acknowledge and thank Ms. Shirley Thornton for reviewing my manuscript and helping with the editing. I want to thank the staff of Balboa Press and Hay House for their professional support and guidance during the publishing process. They have been professional and very helpful.

I also want to thank my granddaughter, Christina, a rhetorical writer, for reviewing this book.

INTRODUCTION

Can you reverse aging and look younger?

Yes, you can. People can live longer and healthier lives if they have a positive attitude and the determination to make changes in their lifestyles. In this book, we will provide a prescription to reverse aging, look younger, and live healthier and longer. You not only can reverse aging, but you can reverse diabetes, heart disease, arthritis, and muscle weakness. You can even prevent cancer.

The prescription is a pragmatic code—or formula—based on my personal experience as a clinician and over forty years of practicing medicine, advising patients on how to maintain a healthier lifestyle. Additionally, my wife and I have lived by this code, and we indeed look much younger than our chronological ages. In this book, we want to share our code to looking younger, living healthier, and enjoying a happier life. What is important for anyone who wants to reverse aging, live longer, and stay healthy is to make a choice, have a positive expectation, and develop the discipline and attitude to be ready physically, mentally, and spiritually for such change while having a goal to be happy along the way.

My wife and I believe that our biological and psychological ages are what matters. It is not the abstract number of chronological age that determines our lives, activities, and happiness. What is meaningful is how our bodies look and function and how healthy and happy we feel as we age gracefully. Although in our seventies, we both feel younger and healthier than when we were in our forties. We can say without hesitation, "We are as old as we feel." We not only look twenty to thirty years younger than people of the same age do, we actually feel healthier. Many of my patients, friends, and family wonder how we do it. They ask us frequently what we eat or do to stay young and healthy. They want to know the "secret" or the "formula." In reality, there is no secret; it is lifestyle that determines whether we feel happy, look younger, and are healthier.

This is the reason for writing this book. It does not matter how wealthy or powerful you are if you cannot make choices to achieve the changes required to reverse aging and live longer. When it becomes clear in your mind that the reason you want to live longer and look younger and healthier is an intense desire to take care of your physical, emotional, and spiritual health and to pursue greater happiness, you are ready for this change.

The first step to realizing these changes is to make your mind the center of creativity and direction. Everything starts when you channel your thoughts and direct them to change your internal and external environment and bring yourself into equilibrium. We will cover this topic more extensively in chapter 1.

Your mind will direct you to make the adjustments and the changes necessary to reach your destination. For example, when women reach an age of menopause and hormones begin to decline, they need to make adjustments to slow down the decline and the symptoms associated with internal changes going on in their bodies. The same is true for men when low testosterone levels cause a gradual decline of their health and libido, which can cause significant consequences if not reversed in time. All this will be explained in more detail in chapter 7, about sexuality.

Nutritional deficiencies, inactivity, poor diets, stress, and insomnia, everywhere in the world, may take a toll as well. We will explain the best diets for healthy living and weight loss and bad diets that may lead to cancer or heart disease more extensively in chapter 2.

The importance of resting and taking a break to enjoy a moment and enhance happiness is explained in chapter 3. The influence of exercise as part of healthy living and prevention of weakness and improved brain function is explained in chapter 4. As we age, we lose strength, and muscles become weaker. But we can compensate for this loss through exercise. We address these issues in more detail in this chapter.

We dedicate chapter 5 to stress, since this universal problem plays an important role in our daily lives. Learning to deal with stress and using meditation to improve our resilience is explained in more detail in this chapter.

The importance of sleep to maintain our health and reverse aging is essential for a healthy lifestyle and is explained in more detail in chapter 6. We address how hormones released during a night of deep and refreshing sleep affect our bodies for healthier living in this chapter. We feel that sexuality and sex are important to achieve love and happiness. This will be explained in chapter 7, where you will find recommendations about hormone therapy and supplements to improve hormonal balance and libido to reach greater happiness.

We couldn't dismiss the importance of spirituality to make our lives whole. In chapter 8, you can find personal events and stories that help to illustrate the importance of spirituality in our lives.

To bring all the brain and body functions into balance, there are steps you can take to reverse aging, prevent illness, and decrease the associated problems of these deficiencies. You will succeed, if you follow the prescription described in this book.

The prescription is summarized with the acronym DRESS-SS, which stands for diet, rest, exercise, sleep, stress management, sexuality, and spirituality. This is a word that is easy to remember and is the code or formula that will guide you to develop a healthier lifestyle, look younger, and live longer anywhere in the world.

The first chapter, about the mind-body connection, is followed by chapters about diet, rest, exercise, sleep, and stress management (DRESS). These are the basics when it comes to reaching your goals. To make the prescription more complete, two additional chapters (SS) are dedicated to sexuality and spirituality. We hope all these chapters become your secret weapon to preventing illness, looking younger, increasing longevity, and living a healthier lifestyle.

In this book, you will also find valuable information to help you lose weight and information on healthy foods to prevent cancer and chronic illness, manage stress, and reverse aging.

To learn more about recent research to improve longevity, genetic technologies, telomere, and DNA discoveries to improve health, we provide extensive information in chapter 9. Our final chapter, 10, is a conclusion to bring all this information together and provide a perspective toward the future of living healthier, longer, and happier lives. Appendixes A and B offer information about herbs, supplements, vitamins, minerals, OTC medicines, and creams, organized by diagnosis of problems encountered by many people. We have included tables that provide a guide to foods rich in antioxidants and low in carbohydrates for healthier eating in chapter 2.

Appendix C offers information about care of hair and skin and some useful products. We also offer information on healthy smoothies and desserts rich in antioxidants, minerals, and good fats (Appendices D and E). Appendix G provides information about affordable online labs for blood, genetic, and telomere testing. We hope this book becomes your best companion anywhere you go.

May love and happiness be with you always,

Jairo A. Puentes, MD
Clara I. Puentes

CHAPTER 1

The Mind and Body Connection

Can Our Minds Influence Our Biological Processes?

Our minds, through our thoughts, help us to make choices. Awareness helps us to change our perspectives and guide us to make the right choices when we are uncertain about what to do or which pathway to follow to reach our desired destination. When our bodies look younger and all our systems are running well and balanced, we are biologically younger than our chronological age. If we feel happy and healthy, we may feel younger, as well. When this happens, our psychological age may be anywhere between our biological and chronological age; or in many instances, we may even feel younger. I can say with certainty that we can change our bodies, feel younger, and reverse aging if we make up our minds to do what is important to reach such a goal. We should keep in mind, along the way, that our long-term goal or destination is greater health and happiness. To achieve this, never substitute or displace greater happiness for little happiness or pleasure. Smoking may give you temporary pleasure, but long-term smoking will cause you to develop heart disease, COPD, or lung cancer. The same is true for alcohol or opioid dependency. The greatest pleasure in life is a healthy body and mind, full of joy, every day of our existence. A healthy mind will help you make the right choices and influence your mental and physiological processes.

The mental process to make these decisions resides in the power of the mind over the body. Our mind power allows us to make choices and decisions and determines where we want to go and what to do. There is no question about the power of the mind to influence the biology of our bodies.

To make good decisions and enjoy life, we need a healthy brain. As we age, our brains experience some loss of mental and cognitive function. Brain cells die because of age and trauma or nutritional deficiencies. Memory loss is the most significant factor that may affect our overall health and happiness. Loss of brain power may become devastating as we age. This fear is always present as we age if we experience temporary memory loss, become forgetful or begin to make frequent mistakes. This is another reason to make changes in our lifestyles—to keep enjoying life to the fullest until the end. The goal is to keep the brain young, healthy, and balanced so that we can experience joy and optimal cognitive function. Brains shrink as we age. This can be prevented by maintaining optimal cognitive function, social skills, daily exercise, proper nutrition, rest, and sleep. When brain size declines, cognitive functions decline as well. When this happens, brain power and processing of neurological transmission diminish, resulting in gradual deterioration of our bodies. Early brain changes are referred to as mild cognitive impairment, or MCI. As these impairments continue, the person affected will eventually develop dementia or Alzheimer's disease. This process may take over twenty years.

The good news is that, if you do something about it and apply my DRESS-SS prescription, you are going to find that your life will change for the better, reversing brain decline and loss of cognitive abilities. You not only be able to preserve your brain power and cognitive function but will be able to strengthen your immune system, delay chronic illnesses, reverse aging, live healthier, and look younger and happy.

How are the brain and body structurally and chemically connected?

Our brains are the most complex and remarkable organs in our bodies. The brain is connected to all the parts of the body through the nerve system.

The nerve system is made up of microscopic wires that connect at different points, carrying electrical impulses generated by chemicals known as neurotransmitters. The brain wiring system is like an alarm system in a home or building complex. The system has receptors that send electrical impulses to a central processing station, which in turn generates a response. The brain's electrical activity begins with a stimulus to a receptor that may be located in the skin, joint, ligament, muscle, or any of the senses. The stimulus could be a thought as well. When the stimulus travels from the periphery where a receptor is stimulated, the nerve impulse is transmitted through a sensory nerve. There are different types of sensory nerves. Some are highly specialized and specific for transmitting pain impulses, temperature changes, joint positioning, muscle activity, tactile sensations, smells, hearing, taste, or vision.

The nerves traveling inside the spine and brain are known as the central nervous system. Those traveling outside are known as the peripheral nervous system. Some nerves specialize to check the blood vessels or internal organs; they are known as the sympathetic and parasympathetic systems. They all play important functions in response to different types of stimuli. The central nervous system contains about a 100 billion neurons. Through neurogenesis, we know today that it is possible to reproduce nerve cells.

The neurons have a body with a nucleus, branches called dendrites, and a long tail or extension called the axon. The neurons connect with other neurons through the dendrites and axons. The command from the nucleus travels as a nerve impulse to stimulate the release of a neurotransmitter at the end of the dendrites or axon. The chemical released has a specific function on the subsequent nerve cell being stimulated. The space between the neurons' endings is called the synaptic gap. The amount of chemicals released helps to modulate the response of the second or subsequent neurons. This is how the brain manages the mind and body functions.

The chemical energy is transformed into electrical energy to continue the process of transmission until the final destination. The brain is always in a constant state of releasing these chemicals to maintain a balance of the mind and body functions.

This is the key for our well-being. When all the chemicals are in balance, we feel healthy and rested. When one of the chemicals is excessive or deficient, the body or the affected organ responds with an overreaction, no function at all, or in an erratic manner causing a dysfunction.

The most important neurotransmitters or chemicals are:

1. Dopamine, a chemical that is closely related to the release of adrenaline – This chemical controls body functions related to power, including blood pressure, metabolism, and digestion. Dopamine generates electricity that controls voluntary movement, intelligence, abstract thoughts, goal setting, and long-term planning.

A decline of dopamine leads to fatigue, loss of attention, addiction, and voluntary movement.

2. Acetylcholine, a chemical that determines brain processing speed – This chemical allows the easy flow of energy and information transmission through the nervous system. High levels of acetylcholine are associated with creativity and a feeling of wellness. A lack of acetylcholine is associated with loss of brain speed, causing "brain fog," which is evident when someone feels his or her thoughts are disjointed. In severe cases, a lack of acetylcholine is linked to dementia and Alzheimer's disease, a type of dementia that occurs when the brain forgets to take care of the body.

3. GABA, also known as gamma-aminobutyric acid – This chemical is connected to electrical balance. It affects stability and calmness. It is the equivalent of Xanax or Valium. GABA provides relief of anxiety, improves mood, and helps the person to make good decisions. GABA is also involved in the production of "endorphins," the feel-good hormones that help to reduce pain. Endorphins are released by stretching, exercise, and sex activity. A deficiency of GABA causes headaches, palpitations, seizures, and anxiety.

4. Serotonin, a chemical connected to synchrony – Serotonin provides a healing and nourishing effect. It makes a person feel happy, with a feeling of satisfaction. When serotonin is balanced, good restful sleep is improved, as well as rational thinking. When levels are low or out of balance, a person feels depressed and complains of insomnia, eating difficulties, and sensory deprivation.

5. All these chemicals are synergistic, related to each other, and are carefully controlled by the brain. A well-balanced individual is expected to have very few deviations from the normal ranges. Dopamine and serotonin work in conjunction with each other. When one is high, the other may be low. Dopamine and acetylcholine work as the "on" switch to provide lots of energy, while GABA and serotonin work as the "off" switch, to provide calmness to the body.

6. When the body is balanced, a person is creative, energetic, and calm; sleeps well; and is able to relax. Extreme releases lead to bipolar disorders, causing a person to fluctuate from one extreme to another.

As we age, the structure of the brain is worn out and the transmission of chemicals becomes deficient. This is when a person may begin to feel less energetic or forgetful or experience a feeling of losing the mind. This is why keeping a youthful mind is so important. Keeping the brain young, healthy and well balanced will delay aging and loss of mental abilities (Braverman 2011, 3–7).

How do hormones influence the brain?

Another system that has a powerful effect on the brain and the body is the hormonal system. Natural hormones are produced by different glands in the body and act as brain and body chemicals. They connect to the brain through the pituitary gland, which in turn send hormones to affect all cells in the body or specific glands. When the system is operating normally and is well balanced, you feel energized, smart, healthy and happy. As you get older, the hormone output declines and the organs begin to lose function. Failure to maintain a proper balance of these chemicals or hormones, will accelerate the aging of an organ and the entire body, leading to different diseases.

Examples of such diseases are hyper or hypothyroidism, hypogonadism, and so on. The brain, in an effort to rejuvenate an organ, sends impulses to the hypothalamus, which in turn contacts the pituitary gland to release a hormone to stimulate the aging organ.

Without a feedback response, the body raises the levels of cortisol, leading to anxiety, brain fog, and increased belly fat. As each organ begins to fail, your overall health begins to decline, including your intellect, memory, and cognition. Hormones affect different aspects of cognition at each developmental stage of life. A person reaches the highest levels of memory and attention just after puberty, which is a time of a dramatic increase of hormone production.

Memory and attention begin to decline with menopause in women and andropause in men. A hormone decline is what makes you feel tired and with mental fog. You also begin to notice that you can't keep up with the young. This is more evident in men as testosterone levels decline leading to erectile dysfunction or ED.

The good news, as will be explained throughout this book, is the ability to rebalance this deficit by bringing back your hormones to optimal levels through hormone replacement. This allows you to be at peak intelligence, top physical shape, and peak performance. Hormone replacement therapy improves brain speed, one the most important functions of the brain in terms of your thinking. By keeping your natural hormones balanced, you will continue to enhance the production of the brain neurotransmitters or brain chemicals.

I usually recommend estrogens and testosterone to women in the form of vaginal creams and testosterone to men, all of which will be discussed in in more detail in chapter 7. I also recommend DHEA, GABA, and other supplements like melatonin. Melatonin has a beneficial effect by helping to increase the levels of growth hormone and serotonin at night (Braverman 2011,195–97).

To maintain top brain and body function, you have to pay attention to the nutrients and foods you consume. What you eat determines the health of your brain and body cells. I will be covering diets, nutrients, and supplements in chapter 2.

How can brain power be improved?

Brain power requires awareness and education to maintain optimal memory and cognitive functions. Developing awareness creates an alert system that helps us to take precautions to prevent problems down the road. You should read books and articles, socialize, exercise, rest, sleep for a sufficient number of hours, and enjoy every moment to enhance brain power. A disciplined lifestyle is very important to maintain your brain and body in balance. It requires a constant awareness of the best foods and behaviors to improve health, a positive attitude, and an intense desire to make the right decisions. Besides awareness and education, we need to be alert and consistently remind ourselves of the consequences of bad behaviors that may affect our health, safety, and longevity. We may still play sports, work, and take risks, but they should be measured risks. Recklessness is not an acceptable behavior because it is destructive and may affect our longevity, happiness, and standard of living.

To improve brain power as you get older, you should be aware of the decline affecting all organs, including the brain, and actions to contain and stop this decline. Your best approach is to follow my prescription, since it provides a balanced approach to improve your brain and body functions. My longevity code is summarized in the acronym DRESS-SS (diet, rest, exercise, sleep, stress management, sexuality, and spirituality). This code is your passcode to enter a new world of wellness and happiness for a better future. Each letter represents an important action to improve your life for greater happiness. I will discuss the meaning of this prescription in more detail in subsequent chapters. You can jump to any of the chapters at any time to address a particular topic that is of interest to you. I'll provide additional information in the appendixes about diet plans, recipes, skin and hair care, supplements, and exercises.

How can negative thoughts and attitudes make people age faster?

There is no question that our minds control our bodies. Mind over matter is a very important concept. Your neurotransmitters and hormones play an important role in your mind and bodies. Excessive release of any of them may lead to illness, and too much stress will damage your organs and overall health. This, in turn, affects the way you look and will be reflected in your face and in the way you stand, walk, sleep, and eat. Negative people look angry and depressed and have a bad attitude. They project bad energy, feelings, and thoughts onto those around them. People low in serotonin have more health problems. Any person who complains about everything is not happy. His or her words and gestures quickly reveal that something is wrong. People under a great deal of stress age more rapidly and are generally unhealthy. They frown more often and have wrinkles on the forehead. Their facial folds are deeper, and their upper eyelids sag. They may have bags under their eyes. They are unable to go into deep and refreshing sleep night after night. They may be dependent on drugs, sleeping aids, or medications that may affect memory and intellect. Because they do not feel well, they may not exercise enough, often feel tired, eat poorly, have nutritional deficits, and gain weight. If they have insomnia, they may drink alcohol, use drugs, or smoke. They usually look older for their age.

You can tell from the negative energy depressed people project that they have problems and most likely are making bad choices. The life spans of people who are depressed or are under constant stress is shortened by illness, a weak immune system, and potential damage to their DNA. The telomeres in their chromosomes shorten with chronic stress, limiting life spans. It is not surprising that people under stress age faster and die sooner than their peers who are less stressed. The wise saying, "You are as old as you feel," applies to them.

But there is hope when people decide to change, meditate, and make positive choices. There is no question, people in these situations can reverse aging and improve their emotional state if they begin to exercise, eat better, sleep better, enjoy life, express gratitude, and again feel the love of those who care for them.

What influence does the mind have on our genes?

We touched before on the influence of the mind over the body. This power goes deeper at our cellular level. When we move a finger, we have to think which finger and which hand will perform the action. A thought begins this process, and a nerve or group of nerve cells in the brain generate a nerve impulse. These nerve impulses travel through the brain, down to the spinal cord, and through the nerves to the muscles. When that impulse reaches the muscle, the muscle fiber gets the order and contracts. If a group of muscles is called into action, all of them in a synchronized manner execute the order, and the finger moves in the desired direction for a specific action.

Imagine a pianist playing beautiful music in a concert. The movements are precise and carefully executed under the control of the mind. The audience enjoys the product of this magnificent mind and body connection. The mind creates or produces the music. The sound that we hear is the product of such a creation. Many nerve cells contribute to these creations. At the genetic level, our chromosomes store the information to be conveyed to our muscles so they can execute a predicted action. Such a creation is stored in files located in memory banks in specialized areas of our brains. All these memory banks and files are interconnected to generate the appropriate action.

Our chromosomes contain the genes responsible for many functions and determine the time cells may stop to divide or stop a cell function. The ending of the chromosome is known as the telomere. Telomeres look like small cuffs at the ends of the chromosomes. The telomeres in our chromosomes determine the longevity of the cells. In 2009, three scientists received the Nobel Prize in Medicine for discovering how the loss of telomeres influences aging, what is now known as the "telomere effect." The telomere's length is controlled by the enzyme telomerase. When the amount of this enzyme is in decline, the cells die quickly. When the levels of this enzyme increase, the telomeres get longer, prolonging the lives of the cells. This seems to explain why some organs begin to age early. Telomere shortening has an effect on our immune system, our cardiovascular system, and essentially on all organs.

The telomere effect demonstrated that women caring for chronically ill children experienced shortening of telomeres when major stressors were present. Some women who exercised and had healthier lifestyles maintained their telomeres' length. It appears that lifestyle changes have an effect on the telomeres. Blackburn and her fellow researchers found that the damage was more frequently present in those with sedentary lifestyles. Their conclusion was that our life experiences and the way we respond to those events could change the lengths of our telomeres. In other words, we can change the way we age at the most elemental cellular level. We now have scientific proof that we can affect our telomeres at the cellular level. These findings are revolutionary. Shortening of telomeres is not limited to the old but can take place in any person regardless of age. We can conclude that a healthy lifestyle prolongs and maintains the telomeres, prolonging life and reversing aging.

This implies that the healthier we are, the healthier our telomeres become, and the possibility of living longer and healthier is real and within our reach. I would not be surprised if, in a few decades, a person with a chronological age of a hundred may look thirty or forty years younger. In other words, this person's biological age may be sixty or seventy. I predict that, within one generation, our biological age will become more relevant than our chronological age. It will be possible to enjoy a longer life span and look half of our chronological age. Anyone planning to keep his or her telomeres healthy should be ready to enjoy more years and, hopefully, a healthier long life. Very likely, stress reduction, good sleep, rest, exercise, proper diet, and proper nutrients and supplements may play a role in increasing the enzyme telomerase at the cellular level, which keeps your telomeres longer and healthy.

My prescription for a healthy and long life

D is for Diet
R is for Rest
E is for Exercise
S is for Sleep
S is for Stress management
S is for Sexuality
S is for Spirituality

This is the code or password for your fountain of health and happiness. Read every chapter and apply my prescription for a better life.

CHAPTER 2

D is for Diet

Never sacrifice greater happiness for little or small happiness.
—Epicurus of Samos

The words of wisdom by the Ancient Greek philosopher Epicurus of Samos that open up this chapter have guided me throughout my life to help me achieve success and greater happiness. Eating is one of greatest pleasures in life, but eating the wrong food or eating in excess can cause harm. Junk foods and sugary drinks may provide immediate gratification, but over the long term, they will cause harm. Children raised with harmful diets that include these things will eventually develop diabetes or heart disease or will die too early as adults. It is better to eat the right kind of food as we grow up, rather than to suffer illness or premature death later in life.

This chapter will cover diets, vitamins, minerals, and supplements in more detail. Since personal health plays a crucial role in these pursuits, we must first address diet and nutrients that are essential for a healthy lifestyle and examine how nutrients and free radicals may affect our chromosomes and mitochondria at the cellular level. Most people understand that food is one of the basic elements necessary to stay alive. However, without proper nourishment, we cannot survive. Poor nutrition is detrimental to our health and leads to nutritional deficiencies at the cellular level and in supportive tissues, which can cause serious health consequences. "Approximately 25%

risk of death is due to genetics and of the remaining 75%, diet is likely the most important factor," says Luigi Fontana a physician and codirector of the longevity research program at Washington University in St. Louis (quoted in Heid and O'Connor 2015).

The Dietary Guidelines for Americans provide guidance based on eating patterns. I will provide more information about the guidelines later in this chapter. I want to make clear that these guidelines, although scientific and based on evidence, change every ten years. They are rather generic and, in many instances, allow too many sugars and fats. I am particularly concerned about the recommendations of fruit juices, sugar, and animal fat intake. I personally feel there should be more restrictions on consumption of sugars, saturated animal fats, and meats, since they are the cause of many health problems.

Nutritional deficiencies start from the moment we are conceived. A mother who is deficient in folic acid will create a deficiency for the fetus that can prevent the fetus from developing a normal nervous system. Most children born with spine defects or brain problems, such as spina bifida, had a deficiency of folic acid in utero. Since your goal is to reach a healthy and long life, women must be aware of these deficiencies. Once a woman gets pregnant, she must educate herself about the potential effects of nutritional deficiencies, drugs, or behaviors that may affect her unborn child. Failure to do this may cause a heartache that will last a lifetime for her and the innocent child.

Once we are born, mother's milk is an excellent food full of essential nutrients and antibodies that protect the child against many illnesses. As children grow and develop, they need more nutrients to help their bodies to grow healthier, and mother's milk may be insufficient to feed a rapidly growing child. Reinforced formula or milk and additional foods must be added to the diet of an infant to prevent nutritional deficiencies. In the infant stage, a child develops good or bad behaviors that may have good or catastrophic effects on his or her overall health and life span. One of the most catastrophic effects in younger generations is the development of obesity. Parents play a big role in the development of obesity in a child. Overfeeding a child, particularly with a diet rich in refined sugars, carbohydrates, and fats, may lead to permanent problems, which will become more apparent and serious as the child enters adulthood.

The negative effects of a wrong diet

Obesity

The major culprit of obesity is the consumption of and addiction to refined sugar. Parents should not use sugary drinks like sodas or juices to feed their children. The amount of refined sugar in a soda is equivalent to ten teaspoons of sugar. Giving a can of soda full of sugar to a child or an adult is like giving them a slow poison, which eventually will cause obesity, diabetes, metabolic syndrome, and other complications, including damage to the nuclear DNA. Excessive amounts of sugar generate excessive amounts of free radicals, which will damage the DNA and mitochondria. My advice to any good parent is to avoid sugary drinks for anybody in your family as much as possible.

This includes so-called fruit juices, which are also loaded with sugars, like fructose and syrups. Avoid them like a plague. People wonder why juices are harmful since they are made of fruits. The reality is that manufacturers add sugars, even though fruits already contain complex sugars, which take longer to absorb. They make these additions to make juices more palatable. I recommend that you buy fresh orange juice that has less than 50 percent sugars or use the real fruit. Squeezing oranges or blending an apple, strawberries, and bananas in a blender to make juice and smoothies is a better choice. Note: The American Academy of Pediatrics recommends not giving fruit juices to children under one year of age since this contributes to the development of obesity.

Eating fruits with moderation is fine. Many scientific studies suggest that eating fruits and vegetables makes people happier and healthier (Longo 2018; Murray 2017). If you are trying to lose weight, eating excessive amounts of fruits may cause you to gain weight. A banana has a high glycemic index and contains complex sugars that take longer to absorb. The amount of sugar in one banana is equivalent to five teaspoons of sugar. If you are on a diet, eating two bananas a day is equivalent to one can of soda a day. That is why people who are trying to lose weight do not lose weight. They feel they are eating the right foods rich in vegetables and fruits but see no change. Fruits provide good nutrients, along with complex carbohydrates, minerals, vitamins, and antioxidants for more energy. These complex carbohydrates take longer to digest and are not absorbed as fast like refined sugars. However, too many fruits with a high glycemic index will make you gain weight. One orange or apple provides enough vitamins and nutrients for a day.

The excessive daily use of carbohydrates, either as refined sugars, flour, bread, alcohol, or syrups, is another contributing factor to obesity, diabetes, and metabolic syndrome. You can still eat foods made of flour or have a glass of wine without serious problems, as long as you consume them with moderation. One or two slices of whole grain bread are sufficient with a meal, rather than a half loaf of white bread. Just as with fruits, when eating carbohydrates, the key is *moderation.* To delay the absorption of these complex carbohydrates, I recommend adding fiber. You may eat a carrot or blend carrots and vegetables in a blender to prepare a shake or a smoothie. You can use Metamucil to increase the fiber content. A tablespoon of Metamucil will add significant fiber and delay the absorption of carbohydrates or sugars.

In my opinion, the most beneficial foods in any diet are vegetables. I am not suggesting that you become a vegetarian. A healthy diet should include poultry, fish, eggs, and nuts. I recommend meat only on occasions and not more than once a month. Most greens are healthful and are rich in vitamins, antioxidants, fiber, and protein. Adding greens to any diet is a way to live healthy and grow stronger for a longer life. Eating veggies every day is a healthy practice. My recommendation is a modified Mediterranean diet, low in pasta, bread, and carbohydrates, as a way to eat healthy foods and control weight.

Two to three veggies a day should be included in a good diet. Unfortunately, most children reject vegetables in their diets. Why? Parents simply fail to introduce them into their diets very early in the child's development. They mistakenly believe that junk food is good to appease their children for good behaviors and use it as a reward. This is a horrible mistake. Hamburgers and French fries and fried foods low in fiber are not good foods to feed a child. A diet associated with soda, ice cream, and pizza is not healthy and will lead to many health problems as the child grows up. Unfortunately, parents give these kinds of foods to their children, and it is food typically found in school cafeterias. When parents give junk food to children to keep them quiet or to reward them for good behaviors, they send the wrong message and fail to help them develop good eating behaviors for a healthy, long life. Junk diets accelerate the development of illnesses predisposed by our genetic code, one of the most common being diabetes. Adding foods with excessive sugars to a diet is like adding more fuel to a fire. Anyone with a genetic predisposition to diabetes or heart disease should avoid junk foods.

Good behaviors start with proper and responsible guidance by parents. Instant gratification for any good deeds with sugary drinks and foods is detrimental. Awareness, education, and discipline are the elements necessary for developing good behaviors. If parents fail to introduce good foods in infancy, it is likely their children will grow up eating harmful junk foods. The consequences will not be immediate but, rather, cumulative over many years. In my many years as a medical doctor, I have seen many men and women dying of heart disease very early in their lives. Unfortunately, obesity in children today is common. Generally, these children can trace their obesity to the learned behaviors from their parents.

A child should learn from his or her parents to appreciate which are the healthy foods. Greens, well cooked or fresh, can be a delicious treat. Using them to prepare shakes or drinks combined with fruits is a way to introduce greens in a child's diet. I do not dispute the value of eating greens. Some people are concerned that veggies do not provide proteins. They are wrong. Greens can provide all the proteins necessary for all body functions, particularly the functions of a growing child. We just need to look at animals feeding from grass only. Cattle develop into big and powerful animals to give us milk and meat to feed our bodies. They do not consume steaks, fish, sugar, sugary drinks, or fatty foods. They are essentially grass eaters that can reach full development without eating the foods we consume every day.

Most greens contain most essential amino acids, minerals, fiber, antioxidants, carotenoids, flavonoids, and a full spectrum of enzymes and minerals required for a healthy life. The goal is to develop a behavior for a diet that combines vegetables and fruits every day of our lives. Veggies are alkaline and help to combat acidosis. An alkaline diet helps to digest foods, improve metabolism, and increase energy. Blending veggies and fruits in a blender is a way to make shakes and juices children and adults enjoy. I frequently recommend these smoothies to my patients who are debilitated by illness or who want to lose weight. Some of my favorite smoothies made of fruits and veggies are listed in Appendix D.

If you prefer, rather than preparing vegetable-based dishes or eating whole fruits and vegetables, you can substitute fruit and vegetable smoothies to help you ingest the recommended daily quota of whole fruit and vegetables. You can make smoothies from many different kinds of fruits and vegetables. Blending fruits and vegetables is a way to get several servings of fruits and vegetables each day. Examples of good fruits for powerful smoothies are apples, blueberries, strawberries, bananas, dried plums, cherry juice extract, grapes, or kiwi. Examples of good vegetables to add are carrots, spinach, kale, celery, and broccoli. Surprisingly, none of these vegetables detract from the taste and flavors.

Commercial smoothies are not good for you. They are loaded with sugars. A good smoothie should be prepared from scratch with fresh fruits and vegetables. These smoothies are rich in antioxidants that help to prevent damage to the DNA. Packaged frozen fruits are acceptable since they can be stored in the freezer to prevent damage of the fruits. You can prepare your own or find them at your local grocery store, ready to be place in the blender. Orange juice squeezed from the fruit is the best. A smoothie should contain at least 3 grams of fiber. You can add flax or psyllium husk (Metamucil) to increase the fiber content. Fiber slows down the absorption of sugar, which leads to weight gain and more abdominal fat. A smoothie should contain protein to be nutritious. You can add protein powder to provide all amino acids necessary for all body functions or to increase muscle mass.

I start my mornings with my "morning essentials," which combines omega-3 and fresh orange juice to provide two essential nutrients our bodies do not make—omega-3 fatty acids and vitamin C. You can find my recipes for this essential drink to start your day along with the best healthy veggie-fruit smoothies for you and your family in Appendix D. These smoothies could be the basis for a healthy diet and a way to lose weight and reduce unwanted fat. Children will enjoy them and will learn to add veggies and fruits to their diets. Appendix E describes some of my favorite desserts. My coconut blueberry yogurt delight is rich in antioxidants and probiotics.

The obesity problem and disease

Obesity is an epidemic spreading across America. Obesity is associated with multiple health problems and complications, such as hypertension, diabetes, atherosclerosis, heart disease, metabolic syndrome, low back pain, arthritis, degeneration of the joints, premature aging, and loss of productivity. People who are obese usually develop insulin resistance and diabetes leading to a metabolic syndrome. Recent research (Taubes 2016, 258–62) indicates that people with insulin resistance and high levels of insulin and insulin growth factor are more likely to develop cancer. This happens because the cells affected begin to modify the way they use sugar for energy through a process of aerobic glycolysis. During this process, insulin and insulin-like growth factor (IGF) allow the cells to utilize large amounts of sugar as a source of energy for rapid proliferation. During this production of large amounts of energy, the cells release free radicals, which cause damage to the mitochondria and the nuclear DNA, leading to mutations and the development of cancer. This suggests that there is a cause-and-effect relationship between elevated sugar levels and the development of cancer (Murray 2017, 68–71).

A diet rich in carbohydrates causes damage, not only at the cellular or organ level but also at the societal level, affecting the individual, the family, personal finances, and the national economy. The costs for the associated medical care are staggering. The cost associated with the loss of productivity and the price for health care adds up to trillions of dollars.

It is hard to believe that all these problems are the result of poor eating habits, lack of proper education, and bad behaviors from childhood. This tragedy is something that could have been prevented at home and school through awareness, education, and discipline.

We all have a life and a body to protect and should learn to live a healthier lifestyle early in childhood. We can correct unhealthy behaviors and lifestyles through education at home and school. We must not continue to ignore the obesity epidemic that is killing people prematurely and affecting their health, longevity, and finances; the cost of healthcare; and their pursuit of happiness.

Diets rich in carbohydrates lead to an unhealthy environment, where the cells are constantly bombarded by free radicals. This polluted environment is worse when a person consumes carbohydrates and refined sugars day and night. No wonder people with these types of diets eventually become sick, develop type 2 diabetes, and become obese. The good news is that this dreadful situation and environment can be reversed. Decreasing and eliminating carbs substantially from diets helps to clean up the pollution and decrease the oxidative process taxing the mitochondria and the cells' functions. When people use less sugar or carbs, they lose weight when the cells begin to utilize their fat deposits as sources of energy. This is evident in those who have had gastric bypasses and can see their blood sugar levels return to normal and see no need of insulin or hypoglycemic agents anymore. In my practice, I recommend what I call a "fast-keto diet" to those trying to lose weight. To lose weight with this diet, a person should stop eating after 6:00 p.m. and start fasting at that point until 8:00 a.m. the following day to have a minimum of fourteen hours of fasting. This period allows the body to switch from carbohydrates as a fuel to fat and ketones. By burning the fat during fasting, fat will be removed from the stored deposits. Fasting can be extended a few more hours for faster results.

Sugar is addictive

Sugar can be addictive. This is the reason many people gain or cannot lose weight. Sugar induces a pleasurable response in the "reward center" in a special nucleus of the brain, in a similar way that nicotine, heroin, cocaine, and alcohol induce pleasurable responses. Sugar also stimulates the release of dopamine, through which the potent effects of other addictive drugs are mediated. As fewer dopamine receptors become available, the need for more sugar becomes more intense to maintain a pleasurable response. This in turn displaces other pleasurable foods or activities like sex. Sugar causes the body to produce insulin to keep blood sugar within a normal range. Excessive amounts of sugar give the cell a signal that more sugar is available and waiting outside the cell membrane. The lack of more receptors creates a resistance to insulin, which allows the transport of sugar inside the cells. The increased blood sugar and high levels of insulin trigger the production of more free radicals, which in turn damage the DNA and may lead to the development of cancer.

The cells to accommodate the excess sugar create more receptors to accept the sugar on the outside. This is what is found in type 2 diabetes. Type 1 diabetes is characterized by the lack of insulin. In type 2 diabetes, the abnormal metabolism of sugar creates a resistance to insulin at the cell level. In the brain, as is the case with narcotics, sugar stimulates the reward centers, leading to addiction. As the levels of insulin increase, the levels of leptin and growth hormone, which regulate energy and appetite, decrease. If the diet continues to be rich in carbohydrates, eventually the production of leptin and growth hormone stops, leading to an uncontrollable appetite, weight gain, obesity, fatigue, and low energy.

To fight these symptoms, a person has to stop consuming sugars to end the addiction. This would help the body return to a normal balance and metabolic equilibrium. During this period, a person may experience symptoms of withdrawal the same way many addicts to narcotics feel when they quit cold turkey. Once leptin and growth hormone levels begin to rise, the appetite and a sensation of fullness comes under control. A person addicted to sugar begins to feel better. The production of dopamine gradually decreases. The cravings for sugary drinks stops, food tastes better, sleep is improved, thirst decreases, and weight begins to drop. At this point, clothes begin to feel loose because the body is beginning to use fat as a source of energy. The feedback mechanisms return because there is now an internal balance when all chemistries and hormones involved in the sugar metabolism cycle are in equilibrium. When this balance is restored, a person who is on a diet begins to lose weight. Cells overwhelmed by an excess of sugar 24-7 create tiredness and a lack of energy. This goes away as fat is removed from the deposits all over the body. The removal of this excess fat is the first step to losing weight and eliminating the addiction to sugars.

To start losing weight, you have to make a choice and a conscious decision to eat properly and healthfully throughout your life. Without a mental decision and determination to lose weight and live a healthier lifestyle, you are going to fail. However, do not get discouraged. Even if you have done your best to watch your diet and exercise but failed, there are still some ways to help you. Your best approach is to have a physical and ask your doctor to do some lab work to check your thyroid, insulin levels, blood sugar, HbA1c, lipid panel, and sex hormones as a base to monitor your health and keep a record of your progress. If you have been faithful to a diet and have not lost weight over a period of six months, you should consider a lap-band or gastric bypass procedure performed by bariatric surgeons. In my experience, people who had these procedures lost significant amounts of weight. For the most part, those who were diabetics no longer use insulin or take any hypoglycemic agents. Most importantly, they feel healthier and happier because they lost a significant amount of weight.

Can excessive sugar intake cause cancer?

Recent research shows that cancer may be related to high sugar and insulin levels. In 2003, epidemiologists from the Centers of Disease Control, led by Eugenia Calle, published an analysis in *The New England Journal of Medicine* reporting that cancer mortality in the United States is clearly associated with obesity and being overweight. Heavy men and women were more likely to die from cancer than were the lean. In 2004, the CDC did an analysis linking cancer to diabetes, particularly pancreatic, colorectal, liver, bladder, and breast cancers. The clue was the finding of cancer in individuals who were not obese but suffered metabolic syndrome and were insulin resistant. The research showed that people with higher levels of insulin and an insulin-like growth factor (IGF) had a greater likelihood of getting cancer.

In 2005, Scottish researchers reported that diabetics who took metformin, a drug used to lower insulin resistance, had significantly lower levels of insulin and a reduced risk of cancer when compared to other diabetics on other medications. These findings suggest that hyperglycemia, high insulin resistance, and the presence of IGF are promoters of cancer. Further research demonstrated that cancer cells are addicted to insulin to survive. In cultures, cancer cells die if no insulin is available. Researchers at the National Cancer Institute found that breast cancer cells are very sensitive to insulin because they had receptors sensitive to insulin, something lacking in healthy breast tissue. Also the tumor cells have three to four times more receptors that are sensitive to IGF.

Researchers like Lewis Cantley and Craig Thompson believe that cancer is as much a metabolic disease as a "proliferative" disease (quoted in Taubes 2016). Genetic mutations are responsible for these changes. Cancer, as a metabolic disease, uses insulin and IGF as promoters through various steps. First, insulin and IGF elevate blood sugar and insulin resistance. This causes the cell to use a mechanism of aerobic glycolysis, similar to what bacteria use in oxygen-poor environments. Once the cancer cells make this conversion, they begin to burn enormous amounts of energy, using glucose as fuel, which allows them to proliferate.

Thompson suggests that, when the cells use large amounts of sugar, they generate large amounts of free radicals, which in turn have the ability to damage the DNA, causing mutations. This new kind of cell, with different ways to utilize energy, has the capacity to proliferate at a fast rate. At about this time, the high insulin and IGF levels signal to the cancer cells to keep proliferating. Researchers are concerned that the high levels of sucrose and fructose in our foods raise the levels of insulin resistance. Since these sugars are difficult to metabolize, they are deposited in the liver, leading to a fatty liver and metabolic syndrome. It appears that whatever causes insulin resistance also increases the likelihood of developing cancer.

Can foods cause inflammation?

The answer is *yes*. Some people who eat excessive amounts of meat or fish develop gout, a disease that causes intense pain and inflammation of the joints. This is due to elevation of uric acid. Meat is rich in purines that produce high levels of uric acid when metabolized. To find out if you have gouty arthritis, ask your doctor for a uric acid level.

In sections that follow, I will present a case about how *lectines* and WGA cause inflammation in the walls of the gut and the lining of the arteries. Prevention of inflammation must be part of our strategy for healthy living. Inflammation is the source of autoimmune disorders in the intestine, joints, arteries, and peripheral nerves. Damage of the peripheral nerves is the cause of peripheral neuropathy. Inflammation of the arteries leads to the formation of plaque that can narrow the arteries and results in subsequent heart attacks.

Many people are also allergic to many foods. For example, gluten causes inflammation of the bowel and severe changes in the gut. Peanuts can also cause severe allergies and even death. Peanuts contain naturally occurring molds that can trigger the immune response, which would then result in inflammation. Lactose can cause diarrhea and cramping due to a deficiency of the enzyme, lactase, which is required to break down lactose, a sugar present in milk. Wheat germ agglutinin (WGA) and *lectines* cause inflammation of the lining of the coronaries leading to atherosclerosis (Guntry 2017, 154–58). Limiting consumption of *lectins* helps to prevent progression of damage to the coronary arteries and intestinal wall.

Prostaglandins, naturally produced in response to injury or infection, also trigger inflammation. Tissues become inflamed in the presence of prostaglandins. White cells release proteolytic enzymes to remove the offending substances, damaging the good tissues. As more enzymes are released by the white cells, swelling or inflammation of the tissues becomes greater. Along with most conditions in which there is swelling or inflammation, there is associated pain. Prostaglandins and inflammation at microscopic levels are responsible for such pain. Many anti-inflammatory drugs, such as ibuprofen, Naprosyn, and Celebrex, block the production of prostaglandins. They are called, NSAIDs (nonsteroidal anti-inflammatory drugs). Steroids are powerful anti-inflammatory drugs that control inflammation. They are only recommended in cases of severe inflammation and for short periods, unless the problem is chronic or severe. They are quite helpful to prevent rejection of transplants and severe allergic reactions.

Is fasting the answer to losing weight and being healthier?

Fasting allows your body to burn fat and lose weight. There is a process to reach this state. When circulating sugar is low, the body enters a fasting phase or state. During this state, the cells utilize glycogen as a source of energy. Glycogen is like an auxiliary tank available as a source of energy when you are low in sugar. Glycogen is stored in muscles and liver. Before you begin to burn fat, your body burns glycogen. The estimated amount of glycogen in this auxiliary tank is about 500 grams, of which 100 grams are stored in the liver and the balance, in the muscles. The amount of energy generated by the stored glycogen is equivalent to about 2,000 calories. It may take two days to use all the glycogen before you begin to burn fat, lose weight, and trim inches from your body. If you are muscular or have consumed a diet rich in carbohydrates, the amount could be higher than that.

In addition, each gram of glycogen is stored with 3 to 4 grams of water, which means that, when the stores are depleted, you will lose this water weight. This is great news for a weight-loss program. Losing 2,000 calories may take a day or two depending on the level of fasting and exercise. Making the transition from burning glycogen to burning fat is the first step to losing fat and, eventually, losing weight. During this phase, it is important not to eat or consume any carbohydrates because it will disrupt the transition to burning fat. It is important to keep carbohydrate consumption to less than 30 grams a day. Your main source of energy during the fat-burning phase is to eat good fats. During this period of adaptation, you will experience hunger and cravings until your glycogen is depleted and your liver begins to produce ketones as an alternative fuel to glucose. Once the period of hunger and cravings passes, you can go for hours between meals without a feeling of hunger. Eating healthy fats like avocado or macadamia nuts helps to calm you hunger signals.

Once you get used to this routine, you will lose weight and inches around your waist. A ketogenic diet to lose weight will decrease your levels of insulin and may help to cure type 2 diabetes. A keto diet is also beneficial to those with history of cancer or who are experiencing cancer (Kalamian 2017).

Patients with cancer should carefully measure their protein intake to about 1 gram per every kilogram of lean body mass to prevent malnutrition. For more information about keto diets for cancer, I recommend the book *Keto for Cancer* by Miriam Kalamian. This book contains excellent information about keto diets and helps to dispel the misinformation of many other fad diets. I will expand on the Ketogenic diet later in this chapter.

Fasting reduces the levels of glucose, insulin, and IGF-1, a hormone associated with the proliferation of cancers. Fasting helps the cells to economize in terms of activities that require lots of energy, cell growth, and proliferation. It also enables them to step up their housekeeping activities by removing residual materials and damaged organelles or mitochondria. This includes dysfunctional mitochondria found in cancer cells. The metabolic theory of cancer presents a strong argument that dysfunctional mitochondria are at the root of the initiation and progression of cancer (Kalamian 2017, 89–90).

Diet recommendations

What is a balanced diet?

To have a balanced diet, we need proteins, fats, carbohydrates, minerals, vitamins, and antioxidants in the appropriate amounts to keep the body healthy and prevent disease. A balanced diet varies depending on your body size, gender, and physical activities. There are guidelines and scientific studies that offer sometimes confusing information. We will discuss some of the controversies in this chapter.

Dietary guidelines

The USDA provides guidelines based on 2,000 calories a day. These guidelines are useful but have been controversial for many years because the people on the Dietary Guidelines Advisory Committee have conflicts of interests and deficient scientific information. In 1977, the United States released the first dietary guidelines recommending less fats and more grains with industrial processed vegetable oils taking the place of most animal fats. This recommendation was made based on a study of 2,467 men who reported identical cause of mortality. These guidelines lacked evidence to support them. Even the new guidelines of 2015 continue to recommend less than 10 percent of calories per day from fats. In the 1980s, the food industry replaced natural fats like butter with harmful trans fats, industrially processed oils, and more refined sugars to allow the food industry to offer more palatable products. In spite of these guidelines, US health has declined, as evidenced by the increased trends of diabetes, obesity, heart disease, and cancer.

It is important to remember that a diet rich in sugars is detrimental to your health. To prevent the production of damaging free radicals, it is better to prevent their formation by avoiding sugars. A good diet should contain about 1 gram of protein for every kilogram of lean body mass. For most people, this ranges from 45 to 55 grams of protein a day divided over three meals, equivalent to about 15 to 20 grams per meal. As for carbs, the net intake shouldn't be higher than 30 grams a day. If you want to lose weight, the intake should be lower. Anyone with cancer should consider a diet containing between 10 to 15 grams of carbs a day. Athletes who are very active should consume from 80 to 100 grams of net carbs a day. Once you know your targets for proteins and carbs, you can determine the amounts of fat in your diet. The kind of fats you select should be the ones known as healthy fats. You should avoid all refined processed vegetable and nut oils. They are pro-inflammatory and contaminated with herbicides and solvents. Fats should include some saturated fats like those found in fish, poultry, and eggs; polyunsaturated fats from nuts and seeds; and monounsaturated fats like avocado and olive oil. Omega-3 is an essential fatty acid that must be included in any diet. The intake of omega-6 should be low since this fatty acid may damage the cellular and mitochondrial membranes. Some people may have difficulty digesting fats, particularly if they have had their gallbladders removed. If this is the case, I recommend digestive enzymes that contain the enzyme lipase. If you have coronary artery disease, watch your fat intake carefully. Always avoid trans fats, since they damage the endothelium of your arteries and may lead to a stroke and heart attacks.

To obtain more information, I recommend reviewing the 2015–2020 Dietary Guidelines for Americans at www.health.gov. Creating each edition of the dietary guidelines is a joint effort of the US Department of Health and Human Services (HHS) and the US Department of Agriculture (USDA). A new edition is published every five years to reflect advancements in scientific knowledge and translate the science that is current at the time into sound food-based guidance to promote health in the United States. The process to develop the dietary guidelines has also evolved to evaluate existing scientific research, development of policy recommendations, and implementation by the federal government of the dietary guidelines in the multiple settings they influence, from home to school to work to community.

Proteins and fats are present in a variety of foods. Meat, poultry, fish, milk, eggs, fruits, and vegetables are the best source of them. Since every person is different, a correct diet for health may vary from person to person and activity level. The best rule of thumb is to follow a diet that is varied that covers all foods groups and is low in undesirable nutrients such as sodium, unhealthy fats, and sugar. With this simple advice, you are well on your way to a healthy body and happier longevity.

Unfortunately, many children do not eat a balanced diet. The same is true for many adults, especially as they age or take medicines to control an illness. Many families feed their children with soda pops and pizza. This is a poor choice. Children grow deficient in many nutrients with these diets. Many girls do not take enough iron and develop anemia as they begin to menstruate. They also are deficient in folate, which can lead to their children having brain defects. Many boys do not take enough calcium or vitamin D and begin to develop osteoporosis. Many adults with medical problems often take medications that limit the absorption of minerals or cause them to lose minerals through their kidneys. Many doctors unfortunately do not address these problems. They pay attention to the medication and possible side effects but never address issues related to absorption or loss of important amino acids or minerals.

For example, people who take diuretics lose not only potassium, but also sodium, magnesium, calcium, zinc, B complex vitamins, vitamin D, and many other nutrients. When the patient returns for a follow-up visit, most doctors fail to check for the nutritional deficiencies that will continue to decline month after month or year after year. The result is more medical problems down the road. A deficiency of magnesium will make this person more susceptible to diabetes, increasing insulin resistance, which can lead to muscle cramps and elevated blood pressure. In women, this poses a risk of blood clots and stroke, osteoporosis, heart arrhythmias, sudden death, obstruction of coronaries due to formation of clots, increased inflammation, anxiety, depression, painful menstrual cramps, migraines, weight gain, leg cramps, and insomnia. These are some of the problems with only one mineral. If we add the other minerals and vitamins, it is no wonder the person is feeling worse.

Most doctors do not pay attention to these deficiencies because they receive little or no training in nutrition and do not realize the consequences and side effects of these nutrients when they are deficient or depleted. If the patient is feeling tired or depressed or is in pain, the doctor often prescribes an antidepressant or a narcotic analgesic, which compounds the problem. Most drugs have a side effect or cause a depletion of these minerals and nutrients. To prevent this, it is wise to take a multivitamin with minerals every day. At least every six months, the patient should ask the doctor to check the most important minerals when symptoms do not go away. In my practice, I recommend that my patients with such symptoms take magnesium (400 mg a day) and vitamin D (1.000 IU twice a day). Most of the time, the treatment is not the pain pill or the antidepressant. It is a replacement of these nutrients and minerals.

Omega-3 is an essential fatty acid our body cannot make, and it is necessary to build tissues, repair cells, build organs, create defenses, strengthen our immune system, protect the heart, and lower triglycerides. It should be included in your diet every day. This nutrient is a basic element for good health. You can find omega-3 in foods like fish, particularly salmon; flax seeds, hemp, and chia; and oil supplements like krill oil. Vitamin C is an essential vitamin our bodies do not make and need daily for optimal body functions. This vitamin is found in citric fruits like orange juice and many vegetables. These are just two of many essential nutrients that keep our bodies in balance and keep us healthy. My wife and I usually start our day with our "morning essential" smoothie made of omega-3 and orange juice and take a B complex vitamin each day that contains all basic minerals and probiotics. I describe the preparation of the smoothie in the Appendix D and provide lists of some of the supplements, herbs, and botanicals I recommend for different conditions or diagnoses. Please note that these supplements and herbs are *additional* to a good balanced diet, not a substitute. You should not use these supplements as the only treatment for a condition. You should talk to your doctor, who can prescribe the best medicines. Supplements help to prevent deficiencies and side effects.

A good balanced diet of proteins, vegetables, and fruits is all we need to achieve good health. Low glycemic fruits are better if you want to restrict your calorie intake or you are diabetic and have high insulin levels. Fruits with low glycemic index (less than 55) are berries, coconuts, avocados, and olives. Fruits with higher glycemic index are bananas, mangoes, and grapes. Don't consume them in excess since they contribute to weight gain. Additional vitamins and other supplements are not always necessary but will not do harm unless they are used in excess.

My wife and I use some supplements on a daily basis because they are beneficial for many functions, help to prevent nutritional deficiencies or inflammation, or are not available in many vegetables or foods. I recommend cinnamon and alpha lipoic acid since they help to lower blood sugar, particularly if you are prediabetic or have a high insulin level. Alpha lipoic acid is also beneficial since it helps to protect against free radicals produced during sugar metabolism. Free radicals cause damage of the nuclear DNA, leading to mutations and cancer. Our diets require antioxidants to suppress the effects from sugar metabolism and the production of free radicals. I have listed in a table which foods are rich in antioxidants to help you make your selections when buying food. These vegetables and fruits prevent damage of your mitochondria and DNA caused by free radicals. This table was prepared by the USDA to provide guidelines to food manufactures in the USA. It is a good idea to use these foods on a regular basis to fight the excesses of free radicals produced during the oxidative process of carbohydrates in the cells and mitochondria. Fighting cancer using foods that are rich in antioxidants is a way to prevent cancer and extend your longevity.

Vitamin B12 is not present in vegetables. Strict vegetarians should take notice of potential B12 deficiencies since vegetables lack vitamin B12. It is wise to add small amounts of cheese or eggs to the diet if meat or fish is not in a vegetarian diet. Supplements are also beneficial in cases where there are nutritional deficiencies because of a poor diet, intestinal problems, inflammation, alcoholism, pregnancy, or chronic illness.

In my practice, I usually recommend that my patients take omega-3, like krill oil, because it helps to lower triglycerides, decreases inflammation, protects the joints and the heart, builds new tissues, and promotes overall good health.

CoQ10, or ubiquinol, is another supplement, which helps to decrease muscle and joint pain associated with the intake of statins used to lower cholesterol. Many physicians prescribe statins to lower cholesterol but fail to tell their patients to take CoQ10 to reduce achy muscles or joints. Statins utilize CoQ10 for their metabolism and depress the amounts available for the mitochondria to do their job efficiently.

Turmeric, a spice in Chinese foods, helps to reduce inflammation and improve mental and heart functions. This spice must be part of the daily diet. Turmeric in a powder form can be sprinkled in cereal, salads, rice, or on any other food. When combined with pepper, it is better absorbed. Many preparations combine turmeric and pepper for better absorption and results. In a recent case report, a woman in England was cured from myeloma after five years of treatment. Myeloma is a deadly form of cancer without an effective cure.

L-arginine is an amino acid that works as a vasodilator and helps to lower blood pressure and keep the heart healthy. It also improves libido, since it raises the levels of nitric oxide. Watermelons are rich in citrullin and arginine, which also help to improve libido in men and women.

There are many other supplements—when combined with good veggies and fruits—that have many beneficial effects and work better than many medicines with minimal or no side effects. The important point is to be selective and use them appropriately. Check the appendixes for smoothies and salads rich in antioxidants.

As we age, a diet of veggies, fruits, fish, omega-3, B complex vitamins, vitamin D, magnesium, zinc, alpha lipoic acid, probiotics, and selective supplements like SAM-e, melatonin, acetyl-l-carnitine, CoQ10, choline, and melatonin create the foundation for a long and healthy life. This combination provides a healthy edge to all of us as we age.

I emphasize again the need to avoid sugar, fructose, sucrose, and any kind of syrups at all cost. They are dangerous at any age but worse as we enter our fifties when more damage can be done to the mitochondria and nuclear DNA by the excess of free radicals produced during the metabolism of these carbohydrates. I also recommend one portion of fish or salmon two or three times a week, poultry once a week and meat only once a month. I recommend nuts, particularly walnuts, Brazilian nuts, pecans, and almonds. All these foods provide healthy fats.

They provide the essential amino acids, vitamins, and some minerals not found in everyday foods. A good basic diet should include supplements to compensate for deficiencies caused by absorption problems, depletions due to medications or illness, inflammation, or other symptoms, such as anxiety, depression, muscle cramps, headaches, and pain. A multivitamin with minerals once a day is a good option to help to maintain enough minerals if the diet is insufficient to compensate for any deficiency.

If you suffer from muscle cramps, this may be secondary to a deficiency of magnesium. I recommend using a magnesium supplement of 400 mg in the evenings. Muscle cramps are also present if you take cholesterol-lowering medicines. Many doctors prescribe these medicines but fail to advise their patients of this problem and what to do if it develops. Using CoQ10 also helps to relieve muscle pain associated with these medicines.

Check table 1 to select foods rich in antioxidants.

Table 1. Foods rich in antioxidants

Rank	Food	Size	Total antioxidant capacity per serving size
1	Small red bean (dried)	half cup	13,727
2	Wild blueberry	1 cup	13,427
3	Red kidney bean (dried)	half cup	13,259
4	Pinto bean	half cup	11,864
5	Blueberry (cultivated)	1 cup	9,019
6	Cranberry	1 cup (whole)	8,983
7	Artichoke (cooked)	1 cup (hearts)	7,904
8	Blackberry	1 cup	7,701
9	Prune	half cup	7,291
10	Raspberry	1 cup	6,058
11	Strawberry	1 cup	5,938
12	Red Delicious apple	1 whole	5,900
13	Granny Smith apple	1 whole	5,381
14	Pecan	1 ounce	5,095
15	Sweet cherry	1 cup	4,873

16	Black plum	1 whole	4,844
17	Russet potato (cooked)	1 whole	4,649
18	Black bean (dried)	half cup	4,181
19	Plum	1 whole	4,118
20	Gala apple	1 whole	3,903

Public information from USDA. Reviewed by Charlotte E Grayson Mathis, MD, 2005 for WebMD.

Diets to be healthier and lose weight

Obesity and diabetes are prevalent throughout the world. Fat accumulates when we consume excessive amounts of carbohydrates. To live healthier and prevent obesity, you should maintain control of the amount of sugars and carbohydrates in your diet. A low-carbohydrate diet with the proper amount of good fats and proteins will help you to lose weight, live longer, and stay healthier. You can also reverse diabetes and prevent cancer, if you keep carbohydrates to a minimum with a modified Mediterranean diet or a keto diet. I will address these diets later in this chapter. If you are not diabetic but have excess weight, you could benefit from these types of diets. Type 2 diabetes potentially may be cured with a keto diet.

As we described before, the USDA nutritional guidelines have allowed, for decades, increased recommendations for carbohydrates in the form of bread, cereals loaded with sugars, and yogurt loaded with sugars, along with recommending very limited intake of good fats. Since 1978, when 5.19 million Americans were diagnosed with diabetes, the number had more than quadruple when 22.3 million were diagnosed in 2013, according to the Centers for Disease Control. *The Journal of the American Medical Association* recently put the number of adults with obesity at 45.6 percent. These numbers are climbing, particularly in the children's population. Many physicians and researchers consider the guidelines flawed and the reason for the huge decline in public health.

The body was designed to run more efficiently on fats than on sugars. Using sugars for energy creates more damaging free radicals. This is not the case with fats. For decades, the American public has been counseled by the media, the government, doctors, and the food industry that what they need to do is to consume less fat and exercise. The reality is that eating high carbs and little fat makes it extremely difficult to lose weight. By eating too many carbs, you produce more insulin, which signals the body to store fat. The official dietary advice is flawed because it creates a system to make Americans fat (Mercola 2017, 16–20).

I have listed in table 2 the kinds of foods that would help you to lose weight and to maintain a normal weight. The list includes fruits, vegetables, nuts, and beverages. All these foods, combined with eggs, fish, and poultry, along with all the vitamins and minerals necessary, will provide for good nutrition. If you are trying to lose weight, I recommend keeping your carb intake to less than 50 grams a day. Beware that fruits contain sugars and, when combined with other foods, will increase your intake of carbohydrates. Stick to one or two fruits only per day, to keep the carb intake low.

Review my list and keep a copy in your wallet for reference. Use the list when you buy groceries or go out to have dinner. Get used to smaller portions and do not buy fruits in excess since you will be tempted to eat more than is allowed to keep your weight down. Remember that any time you eat sugars or carbs, your insulin level rises. High levels of insulin make you gain weight and increase your fat deposits.

Table 2. A low-carb diet for a healthier life and weight loss

Fruits per cup	Vegetables	Nuts and seeds	Beverages
Avocado	Asparagus	Almonds	Almond milk
Blackberries	Beets	Brazil nuts	Coconut milk
Berries 1/2 cup	Broccoli	Cashews	Broth
Blueberries 1/2 cup	Brussels sprouts	Chia	Coffee decaf
Cranberries	Cabbage	Coconuts	Coffee unsweetened
Grapefruit	Carrots	Flaxseed seeds	Tea (unsweetened)
Lemon	Cauliflower	Flaxseed meal	Water
Lime	Celery	Hazelnuts	Soy milk
Raspberries	Cucumber	Macadamia nuts	

Strawberries	Eggplant	Pecans	
	Garlic	Pistachios	
Half an orange	Green beans	Pumpkin seeds	
Half a pear	Kale	Sunflower seeds	
Pineapple, small slice	Mushrooms	Walnuts	
Watermelon, small wedge or 1/2 cup diced	Okra		
	Onions		
	Peppers		
	Pumpkin		
	Salad greens		
	Spinach		
	Tomatoes		
	Zucchini		

Best diet to keep sugar low and to lose weight

Avoid sugars or carbohydrates as much as possible. When you select foods, always choose those with a low-carb content. A food should not contain more than 15 grams of carbohydrates to avoid large releases of insulin by the pancreas. High levels of insulin make you gain weight.

The best diet to keep sugar low and lose weight and keep you healthy is a modified Mediterranean diet, low in pasta, bread, and legumes, with a moderate amounts of fruits, no meat, fish two to three times a week, poultry once a week, and good fats like olive oil and avocado. We never use sugar or consume sugary drinks or juices containing sugars. This is the diet my wife and I use to keep our weight in check.

We also fast as a way to control our weight. We avoid any foods after 6:00 p.m. and don't have breakfast until 8:00 or 9:00 a.m. We fast from twelve to fourteen hours to help the body and cells to do their repair before we have another meal. We also exercise during fasting, early in the morning before breakfast.

Reading the literature, we found that some researchers recommend time restrictive feedings, or TRF, at least twelve hours a day to lose weight. Animal research supports the hypothesis that calorie restriction can extend life. As I said before, when the cells are overloaded by carbohydrates at the mitochondrial level, the oxidative damage done by the breakdown of carbohydrates releases free radicals responsible for the damage to the cells and the mitochondria. Fasting cuts down the amount of oxidative damage or stress to the cells, reducing and reversing aging. This helps to explain why persons who had a lap-band or a gastric bypass procedure lose weight and show improvement of their blood sugars to the point of not needing insulin or hypoglycemic medications. We can conclude that caloric restriction helps to improve or cure type 2 diabetes and cellular damage and reverse aging.

We also restrict food intake during the week after a big meal at a party, if we gain weight after the event, for two or three days. A meal should not contain more than 50 grams of carbohydrates when you combine all foods. If you are trying to lose weight, keep the carb intake below 30 *grams a day*.

A healthy diet should contain proteins, good fats, and some carbs. Take a picture of my tables and keep them with your photos in your iPhone when you go out to buy foods or have dinner. This is a list of healthy fruits, vegetables, nuts, and beverages to keep with you all the time. Refer to this table to buy foods and to remember what is the best substitute at a dinner or when eating out. Besides these foods, I recommend that you eat fish (preferably salmon) and poultry at least two or three times a week. I also recommend eggs once a day and meat occasionally, only once a month. All these foods contain proteins, fats, vitamins, and minerals essential for cell function. I have listed some other popular fruits but only half portions, since they are rich in carbohydrates.

It is important to avoid foods made of flour, breads, whole grains, cupcakes, cakes, sweet potatoes, potatoes, corn, popcorn, tortillas, ice cream, juices, sugar, fructose syrups, and alcohol. You should pay attention to foods containing lectines since they are associated with the cause of atherosclerosis in the coronary arteries and intestinal problems. Use stevia as a sweetener. Many sweeteners like sucralose and aspartame promote the accumulation of fat, leading to weight gain. Recent studies by Dr. Sabyasachi Sen from George Washington University demonstrate sweeteners cause metabolic dysfunction by allowing more sugar to enter the cells, increasing fat formation. His study was presented at the 99th annual meeting of the Endocrine Society in Orlando in 2017.

Keto diets

For some time, it has been found that ketogenic diets (KDs), which are low in carbohydrates (less than 5 percent carbs) and rich in fats are beneficial to children who suffer from epilepsy or seizure disorders. It also helps children with behavioral disorders, autism, type 2 diabetes, and cancer and older adults with Alzheimer's and Parkinson's disease (Romanoski 2018). It appears cells learn how to utilize fats faster as a source of energy, decreasing the oxidative process and the release of harmful free radicals, which act as pollutants around the cells.

Keto diets are becoming popular to help people with cancer. Miriam Kalamian in her book *Keto for Cancer* makes a compelling case to help patients with cancer to benefit from this type of diet. Through fasting or caloric restriction without malnutrition, it is possible to starve the cancer cells from using carbohydrates to continue their uncontrolled reproduction. This metabolic theory of cancer presents a strong argument that dysfunctional mitochondria are at the root cause of initiation and progression of cancer. This recycling mechanism, also known as autophagy, is triggered by nutrient starvation, according to cell biologist Professor Noboru Mizushima (2007).

Keto diets are also helpful to lose weight. The concept is to decrease the intake of carbs by fasting and utilize the glycogen in the liver and muscles before triggering the switch to burn fat and ketones as the main source of fuel for the mitochondria. This is the equivalent of using a generator in case of a power outage. In this case, the generator is powered by fat instead of carbs, as is regularly done by the cells. What is important is not to introduce carbs during fasting but good fats or oils during this phase. When the body begins to use fats, the liver produces ketones to provide a quick form of fuel, since it takes more time to remove fat from their storages in the fat cells. Fasting could be intermittent or extended to lose weight. Keto diets to lose weight may not be indicated for all cancer patients, since they may be strenuous. Any diet regime must be carefully designed and monitored by a dietician or nutritionist with experience in these diets.

Diets to end coronary artery disease and atherosclerosis

Heart disease is a leading cause of death for men and women in the United States. It claims more deaths than all cancers combined. Obstruction of the coronary arteries causes either sudden death or fatal cardiac arrhythmia. Another problem is enlargement of the heart caused by high blood pressure.

People who die suddenly had no prior warning of heart disease. Most of them die prematurely. Lowering cholesterol and reversing plaque formation and atherosclerosis with diet alone and without medicines should be a goal and will be very beneficial for anyone with a family history of heart disease, evidence of coronary artery disease (CAD) due to genetic factors, bad diets, smoking, and sedentary lifestyle.

Reversing heart disease, particularly obstruction of the arteries by plaque, has been elusive, in spite of the intake of cholesterol-lowering drugs and medicines to control hypertension.

Research to find the most effective diets to prevent and reverse CAD continues. For many patients, it is frustrating to hear from their cardiologists that there is very little to be done to reverse atherosclerosis and progression of obstruction of the coronary arteries. It is frightening for many patients to see that, in spite of losing weight, watching their diets, using cholesterol-lowering drugs, and exercising, the progression of coronary artery disease continues. This can be determined by the increased cardiac calcium scores and narrowing of the coronaries with follow-up catheterizations, stent replacements, frequent heart attacks, and bypass surgery. All these measures, although effective, only provide a few more years of relief of the unavoidable progression of atherosclerosis, heart damage and ultimate death.

A well-known example of the progression of CAD is the case of former Vice President Dick Cheney, who had his first heart attack in his late thirties and multiple attacks thereafter, until his heart was so damaged that his only option was a heart transplant. He was lucky he could find a new heart and is still alive. He was a very conscientious person and followed his doctor's advice but couldn't reverse the progression of atherosclerosis.

The reality is that many patients die of heart disease despite the finest medical care. However, there is hope to reverse atherosclerosis.

Joel Fuhrman, MD, in his book *The End of Heart Disease* offers a diet he calls the "Nutritarian diet" to reverse heart disease. This is a book worth reading.

It is clear that the Standard American Diet or (SAD) is not effective to reverse CAD.

In 1995, Dr. Caldwell Esselstyn published research demonstrating the reversal of coronary plaque and CAD in seventeen patients with severe CAD. He subsequently expanded his research and was able to demonstrate the reversal of plaque. The study eliminated oils, animal fat, fish, diary products, and eggs to avoid the formation of trimethylamide oxide (TMAO), an atherogenic compound found in the intestinal flora when consuming animal products. His results were impressive and effective. Many people and researchers find this diet too radical and rigorous. For some people, this diet is difficult to follow. One of the criticisms is the severe restriction of good fats like olive oil, nuts, seeds, and DHA and EPA fat, which may lead to other health problems. Furhman recommends the addition of these good fats to his Nutritarian diet, along with low dosages of EPA and DHA fats to obtain similar results without other health problems due to nutritional deficiencies.

The Pritikin diet is another plant-based diet, which has been very effective to reverse CAD. Pritikin was only forty-one when he was diagnosed with severe CAD. He developed a diet high in fruits and vegetables and low in oil and animal fats, associated with moderate aerobic exercise. His diet was very effective, and after his death in 1985, an independent autopsy revealed his coronary arteries to be in an excellent condition.

The DASH diet (a diet to stop hypertension and heart disease) recommends lower levels of sodium (less than 2,400 mg for a standard diet and less than 1,500 mg for a low-sodium diet), whole grains, vegetables, fruits, animal fat, meat, poultry, and dairy products. It is like the Standard American Diet (SAD) but very low in sodium.

The Nutritarian diet is a vegetarian diet that includes, whole grains, fruits, beans, nuts, and seeds, allowing from 15 to 25 percent of calories from fat. The diet includes flaxseed and chia daily and 200 to 300 mg of DHA and EPA daily, not fish oil.

Dr. Steven Guntry, in his book *The Plant Paradox* raises new questions about the above diets. Dr. Guntry is a heart surgeon who has conducted extensive research on the use of diets and supplements to eliminate heart disease, diabetes, leaky gut syndrome, autoimmune disorders, and many other diseases. *The Plant Paradox* presents a convincing case of the dangers of some foods like *lectins* and WGA (wheat germ agglutinin) lurking on our plates to damage the coronary arteries and the intestinal wall.

One well-known lectin is gluten, but there are more, causing many problems that have been ignored in many other diets. Take the case of whole grains recommended in the other diets. Wheat is the grain that is most used in our diets, and it is not our friend, according to Dr. Guntry. Most grains and legumes contain lectins, which trigger an autoimmune response. Lectins also play a role in the obesity crisis. No wonder many people can't lose weight if their diets are rich in lectins. Lectins behave like insulin, disrupting the normal passage of sugar inside the cells. Then they direct the fat cells to turn sugar into fat, resulting in weight gain and insulin resistance.

Guntry postulates that low-carb diets like Atkins or South Beach initially work because they eliminate carbs. But as soon as carbs are reintroduced, people gain weight. The same is true with the Paleo diet. What all these diets have in common is that they eliminate lectins initially to prevent them from acting like insulin and depositing the fat in the fat cells. When the lectins are reintroduced, they go back to do their job of storing fat again.

Lectins block sugar from getting inside the nerve and muscle cells, interfere with the digestion of proteins, promote inflammation of the mucosal lining of the gut, cross-react with other proteins causing autoimmune responses, interfere with the replication of DNA, and cause atherosclerosis and the formation of plaque. One way to avoid WGAs or lectins is to avoid whole grain bread or whole grain products (Guntry 2017, 41–45).

Guntry also reveals that a lectine-binding sugar, called Neu5Ac, sits in the lining of the arteries and cells in the gut wall. We share this molecule with elephants, also affected by the same problem. Other species, including chimps and gorillas, don't have the ability to make this molecule and don't get atherosclerosis like humans and elephants. They have a molecule that is slightly different, called Neu5Gc, which doesn't bind with grain lectins.

When we consume red meat, which contains Neu5Gc, our immune system recognizes that this molecule is different, and our white cells react by producing antibodies that attach to the lining of our own blood vessels, which has Neu5Ac. This mistaken attack by our immune system damages the lining of our coronaries, leading to the development of atherosclerosis (Guntry 2017, 154–59).

This is another reason to exclude red meats from our diets. Lots of scientific research now points to a diet low in animal fats to extend life and as more favorable to a healthy longevity. We have to become selective with all the fats we consume. Lectin-containing fats prevalent in the American diet, namely soy, cottonseed, sunflower, canola, corn, grape seed, and peanut, all contain high levels of polyunsaturated omega-6 fats, which trigger an inflammatory cascade in the coronary arteries.

Vitamins, minerals, and supplements

Many diets don't have all the minerals and nutrients necessary for good nutrition. There are some vitamins, minerals, and nutrients that are essential for cellular function and are not produced by the body. Essential fatty acids like omega-3 are important to make cell membranes and repair tissues. Vitamin C is another example. It must be consumed every day. The same is true for many minerals, like iodine and iron. Iodine deficiencies cause goiter, and iron deficiencies cause anemia. Folic acid is a vitamin that may be deficient in many women. A deficiency of folic acid in a pregnant woman may cause brain and neurological damage to the unborn child. This is the reason to use vitamins and minerals as a supplement. Parents should become aware that children reared on soda pop, fries, and pizza do not get enough nutrients and vitamins. The same is true for many women during pregnancy. In addition, as a person ages, most cells do not get enough nutrients due to medications, absorption problems, or bad diets. To be in balance and play it safe, it is better to take a multivitamin with minerals every day.

Many over-the-counter (OTC) medications deplete many nutrients. Aspirin depletes iron, folic acid, vitamin C, and potassium. NSAIDs deplete DHEA, folic acid, melatonin, and zinc. Common prescription drugs, like statin drugs used to lower cholesterol, deplete CoQ10 and vitamins D and E. Corticosteroids, usually taken for inflammation, deplete calcium, magnesium, zinc, selenium, potassium, DHEA, vitamins C and D, and folic acid. Contraceptives deplete B complex vitamins, magnesium, zinc, tyrosine, and vitamin C. In the paragraphs that follow, I will describe in more detail the vitamins' properties, as well as the interaction and side effects of some vitamins and minerals.

Vitamin and supplement uses and interactions

Some foods enhance or decrease the absorption of vitamins. Lectins like gluten, WGA, present in wheat, legumes, and whole grains may cause inflammation of the gut, affecting the absorption of minerals, vitamins, and other nutrients.

Too much calcium can impair the absorption of iron, while vitamin C, for example, increases it. Calcium and magnesium compete for absorption. It is better to take them separately. I recommend taking 400 mg of magnesium in the evening or before going to sleep. It helps the body to relax. B complex vitamins are water soluble, so it is better to take them in the morning. The fat-soluble vitamins (A, D, E, and K) can be taken with meals. Other supplements, can be taken before breakfast or two hours apart from meals.

In Appendix D, I have listed my morning essential that contains vitamin C and omega-3 in the form of a smoothie. You can add other nutrients while you take this delicious smoothie. I usually take my B complex, CoQ10, alpha lipoic acid, and L-arginine with this smoothie. If you establish a routine, you will not miss your daily supplements.

Years ago, my wife developed swelling of the joints of both hands. After trying different treatments, she found a combination of supplements that relieved the swelling. My wife now takes turmeric (curcumin caps), glucosamine, SAM-e, and bromelia to decrease inflammation of the joints of her hands. She found this combination the best to control persistent pain and swelling of her hands.

After this experience, I began to recommend a combination of these nutrients and supplements to my patients, with good results. Many people are unaware of the analgesic and anti-inflammatory benefits of supplements. The FDA prohibits advertising the benefits of supplements because they don't meet the rigorous testing of many pharmaceuticals. The fact is that many supplements have been around for thousands of years, and many pharmaceuticals are made from synthetic chemicals that provide similar beneficial effects of the natural chemicals found in many herbs and supplements. In my experience, many supplements alone or in combination are beneficial to relieve inflammation and pain. As an example, omega-3, SAM-e, and turmeric combined are very safe and good pain relievers.

If you feel you are deficient in any nutrient or vitamin, you should ask your doctor to do a test. Many national laboratories offer tests for minerals and vitamins. Unfortunately, many doctors are simply not trained—or interested—in nutrition and the effects medications cause when it comes to the absorption of nutrients and minerals. Their focus is the prescribed medication and not the disruption of the balance of nutrients, vitamins, and minerals at the cellular level.

If you are tired or without energy, many doctors prefer to give you an antidepressant, when the problem could be low magnesium or vitamin D deficiency. Fortunately, there are labs today where you can get your lab work without a doctor's prescription.

You can find in Appendix G a list of laboratories that offer testing for all these minerals and vitamins, as well as genetic testing when contacted directly. If any test is abnormal and your doctor shows no interest, you should look for a doctor who may be interested in nutritional deficiencies or hormone problems. Searching the internet, you will find doctors in your area who you can contact to address specific problems. Doctors who specialize in comprehensive integrative or alternative medicine offer counseling in nutrition and alternative forms of treatment.

Look always for fresh vegetables and fruits. Fruits and vegetables contain phytochemicals that protect against cancer, heart disease, and many chronic diseases. Among the most potent phytochemicals are pigments such as chlorophyll, carotene, and flavonoids found in a rainbow assortment of fruits and vegetables. Other phytochemicals include, dietary fiber, enzymes, oils, and vitamin-like compounds.

Phytochemicals work in harmony with essential nutrients such as vitamin C, vitamin E, B complex vitamins, zinc, selenium, omega-3 fatty acids, CoQ10, and many other compounds to exert considerably greater protection. They also work as antioxidants to protect against oxidative damage from free radicals that are responsible for DNA damage. Ironically, the major source of free radicals and oxidative damage in the body is the oxygen molecule. The molecule that gives us life is also the molecule that can cause the most harm. Oxidative and free radical damage is the major cause of aging and is also linked to the development of cancers, heart disease, cataracts, Alzheimer's disease, arthritis, and many other degenerative diseases.

The environment also contributes greatly to the free radical load that damages the cells. Cigarette smoking increases greatly the free radical load that causes significant damage. The harmful effects of smoking are related to the high levels of free radicals inhaled, depleting key antioxidants such as vitamin C and beta-carotene. Other external sources of free radicals include ionizing radiation, drugs, air pollutants, pesticides, anesthetics, aromatic hydrocarbons, fried foods, solvents, alcohol, formaldehyde, and many other products used in the home and food processing.

All humans are constantly bombarded by these free radicals and should find protection with a diet rich in vegetables and fruits. The antioxidants in plant foods protect us against free radicals and oxidative damage. Taking supplements can help to fight the damage done by these free radicals.

Vitamin A

Vitamin A is good for your vision and for activating the immune system. Activated vitamin A turns into retinol, which is used in creams to reduce wrinkles. Using these creams during the day is not recommended, since retinol may accelerate the development of skin cancer when exposed to the sun. Some prescription drugs for acne (Accutane) and psoriasis (Soriatane) contain synthetic forms of retinol and are very dangerous during pregnancy because it can cause birth defects. In the bones, retinol integrates with iron and hemoglobin to carry oxygen to the cells.

Too much vitamin A may be harmful for people who smoke, since it predisposes some people to lung cancer. Studies on people who take high doses of beta-carotene or vitamin A show a 28 percent increase in the rate of lung cancer. The death rate from heart disease increases to 17 percent with beta-carotenes.

Another cancer associated with the intake of beta-carotene is prostate cancer. Several studies find an association of increased mortality rate with beta-carotene supplementation. I do not recommend vitamin A if you eat a healthy diet that contains carotenes, which are present in colorful fruits and vegetables. A multivitamin containing no more than 5,000 IU of vitamin A is safe. Pregnant women should not take more than 3,000 IU a day.

Table 3. B complex vitamins

Vitamin B1	Thiamine	Involved in metabolism of sugars and amino acids	Present in whole grains, brown rice, whole green diets, poultry, fish, eggs, pork, shellfish, wheat pasta, yeast, peas
Vitamin B2	Riboflavin	Cofactor of flavoprotein reactions and vitamins	Present in yeast extract, whole grains, liver, cheese
Vitamin B3	Niacin	Precursor of NAD and NADP for many metabolic processes	Present in lean meat, whole grains, brewer's yeast, cheese, fish, eggs, whole wheat bread

Vitamin B5	Pantothenic acid	Precursor of coenzyme A and other molecules	Present in brewer's yeast, royal jelly, liver, nuts, whole grains, eggs
Vitamin B6	Pyridoxine	Coenzyme of many metabolic reactions	Present in wheat germ, bananas, chicken, fish, potatoes, Brussels sprouts, whole wheat bread, green vegetables
Vitamin B7	Biotin	Involved in fatty acids synthesis and gluconeogenesis	Present in peanuts, almonds, eggs yolks, walnuts, chicken, sesame seeds
Vitamin B9	Folic acid	Precursor to make and repair DNA; helps cell division and growth during pregnancy	Present in green diets, poultry, fish, eggs, pork, shellfish
Vitamin B12	Cobalamins, cyanocobalamins, and methylcobalamins	Involved in metabolism of all cells, affecting DNA synthesis and regulation; also involved in fatty acid and amino acid metabolism	Present in liver, beef, pork, fish, eggs, yeast, milk; not found in plants, and vegans may develop a deficiency

B complex vitamins

These are my favorite vitamins. Several vitamins are in this group. They work synergistically to protect the cardiovascular and nervous systems. I have listed them in table 3 with information about their actions. B6, B12, and

B9 are involved in formation of red cells. They also protect the heart against the actions of homocysteine. Most vegetables and fruits have these vitamins, except for B12. Vegetarians who do not consume eggs, fish, or animal food are deficient in this important vitamin.

Folic acid or vitamin 9 is described in more detail below since a deficiency of this vitamin in pregnant women can lead to brain damage of the child.

Folic acid or B9

A green diet is rich in folic acid, and there is no need for supplementation. Poultry, shellfish, eggs, and pork are rich in folic acid as well. It is important to remember that, in just a few weeks, the lack of folic acid in our diet will cause a deficiency. Pregnant women with low folate levels need folate supplementation to prevent defects of the brain, spinal cord, and spinal canal in the unborn child.

Folic acid also helps to decrease the levels of homocysteine, an amino acid responsible for increasing the risk factors for heart disease. A deficiency of folic acid also leads to anemia, loss of cognitive function in children and the elderly, hearing loss in the elderly, skin patches like vitiligo, and slow growth in children.

Deficiencies also develop with malabsorption syndromes like Crohn's disease, celiac syndrome, alcoholism, and kidney dialysis. It affects medication intake of Dilantin, methotrexate, and sulfa.

The required supplemental dose for pregnant women is 400 mcg a day. A pregnant woman should take extra supplementation to protect her child.

Vitamin D

Vitamin D deficiency is a real problem in areas of the country where there is little exposure to the sun. In tropical countries, a few minutes of sunlight increases the levels of vitamin D significantly, while in northern countries or states, away from the equator, particularly during the winter, the lack of sunlight reduces the levels of vitamin D, predisposing people to many illnesses. For most people living in these areas, 2,000 IU of vitamin D is appropriate. In areas where there is more sun, I recommend 1,000 IU once or twice a day depending on the person's level of Vitamin D. If the blood level of vitamin D3 is below 30 mg/ml, a vitamin D3 supplementation is recommended. Good food sources of vitamin D are milk, orange juice, fish, salmon, sardines, fish liver oils, eggs, beef, and butter. Some studies have found an association between multiple sclerosis (MS) and neuromuscular diseases and deficiencies of vitamin D.

There are many other diseases and health problems associated with deficiencies of vitamin D. They include osteomalacia and bone deformities in children, atopic dermatitis, inflammatory bowel disease, asthmatic attacks, cardiovascular problems, sudden cardiac death, cancer of the pancreas, fertility problems, and low testosterone in men with erectile dysfunction. Vitamin D affects about three thousand genes and plays an important role in preventing many health problems and maintaining optimal health. A low level of 25-hydroxy vitamin D is associated with erectile dysfunction, hypogonadism, and fertility problems in hypogonadal men.

Vitamin D also raises the levels of estradiol in men and women and helps to prevent osteoporosis by increasing bone mass. Currently, there are some ongoing studies about the use of vitamin D in the prevention of cancer of the pancreas. Sunscreen decreases the production of vitamin D; a cream with SPF of 8 can lower the production of vitamin D by 95 percent. You need to achieve a balance, since sunscreen protects against damaging UV rays that cause skin cancer and wrinkles. I recommend that you have your levels of vitamin D checked by a doctor to see if you are deficient in this very important vitamin. If you are, you may then consider vitamin D supplementation.

Vitamin E

Vitamin E is an essential nutrient that helps to maintain health and function of the reproductive, vascular, and neuromuscular systems. This vitamin is a great antioxidant and reduces the damage caused by free radicals. Vitamin E helps to prevent damage of the DNA due to oxidative stress. Since inflammation is associated with cardiovascular problems, diabetes, arthritis, and cancer, supplementation with vitamin E in the form of alpha-tocopherol and gamma-tocopherol significantly helps to reduce inflammation.

Many scientific studies confirm these findings. The American Cancer Society, in a study of more than a million adults, found that those who regularly take 200 IU of vitamin E each day have a lower risk of developing bladder cancer. Another study, the SELECT (Selenium and Vitamin E Cancer Prevention Trial), looked at 35,000 men taking 400 IU of vitamin E and found that there is an increase of prostate cancer. For this reason, it is better not to take more than 200 IU of vitamin E (NIH Office of Dietary Supplements 2018).

In a study conducted on veterans at numerous VA centers, vitamin E has been found to decrease the development of dementia and Alzheimer's disease and the decline in cognitive function as we age. Women going through menopause and experiencing hot flashes who take between 600 and 800 IU of vitamin E had significant benefits. Several studies cite the benefits of vitamin E to improve fertility in males. Vitamin E is important to maintain healthy skin, hair, and nails. This is why it is present in many creams and lotions (LowDog 2016, 134–40).

The best sources of vitamin E are sunflower seeds, almonds, spinach, fish, eggs, avocados, green leafy vegetables, vegetable oils, olive oil, and wheat germ.

Prolonged deficiency of vitamin E may increase the risk of peripheral neuropathy, infection, anemia, and problems for the mother and baby during pregnancy. A multivitamin that provides at least 30 IU of vitamin E is adequate. In general, dosages greater than 100 IU are not necessary with a proper diet. Because vitamin E is dependent on selenium, copper, zinc, and manganese, supplementation with these minerals is recommended.

Some individuals, especially those with Crohn's disease, cystic fibrosis, or a genetic disorder known as abetalipoproteinemia that affects the absorption of dietary fats, cholesterol, and fat-soluble vitamins, must take vitamin E supplementation.

Vitamin K

Vitamin K deficiency causes symptoms such as bleeding of the gums, nosebleeds, easy bruising, and heavy menstrual periods. Alcoholics are at higher risk of a vitamin K deficiency, as are people with digestive disorders in which fats are poorly absorbed, as is the case in Crohn's disease, cystic fibrosis, and other intestinal disorders. A diet rich in green leafy vegetables offers a good source of vitamin K. A cup of kale provides 1,000 mcg of K1, while spinach, lettuce, turnip greens, avocado, cheeses, and kiwi fruits help to raise the levels of vitamin K to carboxylate osteocalcin, which can improve bone quality.

If supplementation is required, a dose from 150 to 300 mcg a day is adequate. The dosage of K2 as MK-4 is 500 mcg per day. The subtypes MK-4 and MK-7 are the best for human health. Supplementation can be effective in reducing plaques in coronary arteries. Taking MK-7 for six months lowers plaques and calcium scores. K2 supplementation is important if you have cardiovascular disease, diabetes, or are at risk of osteoporosis or prostate cancer.

Vitamin K2 also helps move calcium to the proper areas of the body. A deficiency of vitamin K2 is the possible cause of calcification of the arteries. The Rotterdam study of 7,983 men and women found that K2, but not K1, has a strong protective effect. There was a reduction of arterial calcification and death when the subjects ate foods rich in K2. Two famous longitudinal studies, the Nurses' Health Study and the Framingham Heart Study, found that people with low dietary intake of vitamin K have greater risk of hip fractures. The lack of carboxylation of this bone-building protein, osteocalcin, is at the root of the fractures. K1 and K2 increase carboxylation of osteocalcin, making bones stronger. Research shows that taking vitamins K and D, calcium, and magnesium helps to keep bones stronger and prevents osteopenia and osteoporosis. However, a person taking warfarin (Coumadin) to prevent blood clots should avoid supplementation of this vitamin.

Minerals

Minerals are elements necessary for many chemical reactions to allow many cells to carry out their metabolic functions. Besides amino acids, vitamins, and other chemicals, cells need minerals to complete their jobs. This is not different than a manufacturer who needs different elements like gold, silver, or copper to finish a product. A lack of one or two elements may produce an inferior product, resulting eventually in a defective outcome. Most vegetables and fruits contain enough minerals in a balanced diet. I am listing the most important minerals for better health below. As far as minerals, I do not recommend the extra intake of iron unless you are anemic or pregnant or have low thyroid and testing indicates you are deficient in iron. Too much iron may be toxic. The same is true with some other minerals.

Copper

Copper is another mineral that should be used with caution. It may reduce the immune function and increase mental decline. It is useful to transport iron to the bone marrow to make red cells. When copper is low, iron accumulates in the liver. A basic multivitamin with minerals provides adequate amounts of copper and other minerals.

Selenium

Selenium is a mineral that is necessary in trace amounts. It is helpful to carry out a number of metabolic and antioxidant processes. This is another mineral that, taken in excess, may be toxic. Selenium is involved in antioxidant reactions to protect the DNA from damage. It is also involved in the production of T-cells, which destroy cells that have been damaged by viruses or bacteria or have become cancerous. Selenium is also involved in the production of thyroid hormones, like T3.

Selenium deficiency increases the risk of viral infections. Supplementation of selenium helps prevent people infected with the hepatitis B and C virus from developing liver cancer.

Low levels of selenium have been associated with higher risks of lung, stomach, colorectal, and prostate cancer. Selenium and iodine are specially related. A deficiency of iodine may worsen hypothyroidism with additional supplementation of selenium.

Selenium is important for reproduction in men and women. Selenium and zinc are important for the production of testosterone and the development of sperm. Low levels of selenium are associated with decreased male fertility and first-trimester miscarriages in women.

Selenium is found in Brazil nuts, shrimp, crabmeat, salmon, pork, chicken, beef, whole grains, garlic, onions, and leeks. A dosage of 100 mcg per day is safe as a supplement.

Calcium

Calcium is an important mineral involved in many functions of all cells. It helps to keep bones strong and teeth healthy. It is important for muscle and nerve function, heart function, and clotting of blood. Calcium from vegetable sources is better. Calcium from stones or mineral sources is responsible for the formation of plaque and stones. Calcium intake protects against lead toxicity by decreasing absorption of lead in the water or foods. A diet rich in fruits, vegetables, poultry, and milk products usually provides enough calcium for the average person. Pregnant women, however, should get enough calcium to reduce the risk of preeclampsia and to help her baby's bones to develop properly. If you take calcium supplements, I recommend no more than 500 mg a day.

Too much calcium in the diet or through supplements may impair the absorption of other important minerals and can even be harmful. It can cause kidney stones and may contribute to hardening of the arteries. For example, if you take calcium to combat osteoporosis, you also need to take vitamins D and K, magnesium, iron, and zinc. Combined preparations of these minerals are available. Calcium alone without vitamin D will not help to prevent osteoporosis. I recommend taking your magnesium in the evening or before going to bed at night.

Chromium

This mineral plays a role in keeping blood sugar levels stable. You only need traces of this mineral. Chromium exists in two forms. The trivalent form is found in food and is necessary for biological functions. The industrial form is hexavalent and is toxic if consumed. The only type of chromium that is safe is the one found in natural foods and supplements. You should never try the industrial form. Vitamin C and some B vitamins are needed to absorb chromium in the gut. This is another reason for using a daily multivitamin with minerals. Research suggests that chromium helps decrease binge eating and weight gain. Chromium allows insulin to enter the cells, making them more sensitive to insulin and helping to maintain good normal levels of blood sugar. Chromium also helps to lower triglycerides and raise good cholesterol or HDL in those taking beta-blockers. Chromium is helpful to control and improve acne and insulin resistance.

Brewer's yeast is a good source of biologically active chromium and more effective than chromium supplements. Meat, eggs, tomatoes, green beans, nuts, whole grains, and meats are good sources of chromium.

Consuming highly refined and processed foods increases the excretion of chromium. People with inflammatory bowel disease may be low in chromium.

Chromium picolinate is the most common form of supplementation. A dose of 120 mcg a day is sufficient for most people. Prediabetics; type 2 diabetics; people with absorption problems, acne, low HDL, or high triglycerides; those who are taking beta-blockers; and many athletes may have higher requirements, with a target dosage of 400 mcg per day. Chromium picolinate combined with vitamin C and 2 mg of biotin per day is absorbed better to improve blood glucose and cholesterol levels in type 2 diabetics and prediabetics.

Iodine

Iodine is a mineral that is essential to produce thyroid hormone. Without iodine, a person develops hypothyroidism. People who are deficient in thyroid hormone gain weight, become obese, and feel tired. They also may have dry skin, muscle cramps, fatigue, intolerance to cold, puffy eyes, constipation, poor memory, and slow thinking. Diets that exclude iodine salt, seafood, and dairy products often lead to lower levels of iodine.

Vegans are at risk of developing iodine deficiency. The Oxford Vegetarian Study found similar results with vegans in the United Kingdom. This may be because of the marginal iodine intake and the higher intake of vegetables that are goitrogenic. Most cruciferous vegetables are goitrogenics. They include arugula, bok choy, broccoli, Brussels sprouts, cabbage, cauliflower, kale, collard greens, mustard greens, turnips, and watercress. The goitrogenic effect in these vegetables has no impact if the diet contains significant iodine levels.

Another factor to consider is the use of chemicals like bromide to purify whirlpools and as a pesticide in fruits like strawberries. Bromide displaces iodine from its receptors leading to iodine deficiencies. Baked foods contain potassium bromide, and some sodas have brominated vegetable oils. Other chemicals that may affect the levels of iodine and the production of thyroid hormone are perchlorate, thiocyanate, nitrate, and phthalate. In a controlled antenatal thyroid study in the United Kingdom and Turin, Italy, from 2002 to 2006, 21,846 women who were less than sixteen weeks pregnant were tested. Perchlorate was detected in all the women and their iodine levels were low. Women with high perchlorate levels have a 300 percent increase in odds of having babies with low IQ at three years of age. Since perchlorate is stored in the mammary glands, it can potentially decrease the levels of iodine in their babies.

The daily requirements of iodine are 150 mcg for men and women. These requirements are higher during pregnancy and breastfeeding. The American Thyroid Association and the Endocrine Society recommend a multivitamin mineral supplement that contains 150 mcg of potassium iodide / iodine daily. This dosage should continue during breastfeeding to ensure the iodine is passed from the breast milk to the baby.

During pregnancy, thyroid hormone is important for the development of the nerves and brain in the baby. Iodine deficiency during pregnancy is associated with high incidences of attention deficit disorder (ADHD), lower IQs, and mental retardation. The World Health Organization (WHO) found that iodine deficiency is the number one cause of cognitive deficiency in children. WHO estimates that over 30 percent of the world population, or more than 2.3 billion people, do not get sufficient iodine.

Fortunately, iodine is found in salt. Sea salt doesn't contain enough iodine. You must buy iodized table salt or iodized sea salt. You may want to eat seaweed, which contains iodine. Remember that the salt used in fast foods is not iodized and is not helpful in producing thyroid hormone. Salt left in a shaker for more than four weeks loses 40 percent of its iodine when exposed to the air. This may result in iodine deficiency and hypothyroidism. People on low salt diets do not get the adequate amount of iodine and will develop hypothyroidism. I recommend they take a multivitamin with minerals that contains 150 mcg of iodine or add seaweed to their diets.

Low levels of iodine can be exacerbated by low iron levels. This is especially true in women who are pregnant. Therefore, pregnant women should take a multivitamin that contains at least 150 mcg of iodine and iron. Both, iron and iodine are essential in the process of making the thyroid hormone. In the United States, roughly 99 percent of processed foods do not contain iodine. People on low-salt diets or diuretics suffer from iodine deficiencies. Hispanic and black women often have the highest deficits of iron and iodine and could have children with mental deficiencies. This tragedy can be prevented by taking vitamins that contain iodine and iron during pregnancy and breastfeeding.

Good sources of iodine are fish, shellfish, eggs, and seaweed. Seaweed has the highest levels of highly bioavailable iodine and is the top food source of iodine. Iodized table salt loses iodine within two months of opening the package. WHO recommends ionization with potassium iodate, due to greater stability, particularly in humid and tropical areas.

Any diet deficient in iron, iodine, zinc, and magnesium most likely will lead to health problems. Iron is part of thyroid peroxidase enzyme, which is necessary to make thyroid hormones. Hair loss, or alopecia areata, may be one early sign of iodine deficiency. Combined with iron, iodine is necessary to provide strength to the hair. If you are losing hair, gaining weight, experiencing an enlarged thyroid gland, or suspect you are at a higher risk of having children with mental retardation, ask your doctor to run blood tests to check for deficiencies in T3, T4, T7, TSH, serum ferritin levels, TBIC (total iron-binding capacity), zinc, and magnesium.

Since my prescription for healthy living is to help you live longer and reach your final destination in optimal health, you should have these tests as part of a yearly physical as you age. If you begin to develop any of the symptoms noted above, ask your doctor or order the test from labs that do not require a doctor's order and are listed in the resources section.

Iron

Iron is a mineral that, according to WHO, is the most deficient nutrient in the world. Iron is found in both animal and plant foods. This deficiency is staggering in developing nations and is usually associated with parasitic infections, malaria, and TB. Iron deficiency anemia contributes to about 20 percent of all maternal deaths in the world. Anemia in the mother contributes to premature and low birth weight, which will impair the child's cognitive and behavioral development. In my opinion, vitamins with iron and minerals should be given free to all women all over the world during pregnancy and lactation. Taking too much iron for too long may be dangerous. If a person has no anemia and iron levels are normal, there is no need for additional iron. Iron can be toxic when taken in excess. Iron can accumulate in all organs, causing damage to the liver, pancreas, heart, and brain. The only solution for too much iron in the body is to donate blood regularly and avoid taking additional iron. It is always wise to use iron only under the direction of a doctor.

Iron deficiency develops from low dietary intake, poor absorption, or blood loss. In my practice, I find people who complain of easy fatigue or weakness and dizziness to sometimes be anemic. Usually the first question is to wonder why this is happening. In women, excessive loss of blood during menstruation or gastrointestinal bleeding by stomach ulcers or hemorrhoids may be the cause. A complete blood test and differential, CBC, is an important test. Other causes may be a diet deficient in iron or poor iron absorption. Anemia may be also caused by deficiencies of vitamin B12 or folic acid. It is very important to see a doctor if you are anemic or losing too much blood.

Iron is necessary to make hemoglobin, the protein in the red cells responsible for carrying the oxygen to the tissues. More than 60 per cent of our iron is in the hemoglobin. Iron is also present in myoglobin, a protein in the muscles to provide sufficient oxygen to hardworking muscles.

When iron is low, hemoglobin levels drop, as does oxygen to the tissues.

With less oxygen, the tissues can't carry out their metabolic functions and produce energy. Without enough oxygen, the muscles can't do their jobs, and a person feels weak. The brain without enough oxygen is affected. A lack of oxygen to the brain causes dizziness and lack of attention and concentration.

Anemic children are unable to concentrate and learn anything in school. Some doctors and counselors recommend psychostimulants to children to improve their concentration when the real problem is anemia and treatment of nutritional deficiencies, including iron. Parents must request a CBC, a complete nutritional assessment, and iron levels before they consider any psychostimulants.

The daily recommended allowance of iron is 8 mg for men and 18 mg for women from ages nineteen to fifty. After menopause, the requirement drops to 8 mg for women. During pregnancy, the requirement is 27 mg per day and 9 mg during breastfeeding.

Vegetarians should double these minimum requirements.

There are two forms of iron found in food—the heme and the nonheme. Meat contains both forms, while plants contain only the nonheme iron.

We absorb only 18 percent of the heme iron and 10 percent of the nonheme. This nonheme could go down to 2 percent in a vegetarian eating mostly beans, rice, grains, soybeans, and lentils, due to a compound in these foods called phytic acid that reduces the absorption of iron.

The absorption can be increased by legumes with vitamin C. Another way to increase the absorption of nonheme iron is to add chili peppers, which are a great source of vitamin C. Eat shellfish and nuts; dried foods and fortified foods are also a good source of iron, as is cooked spinach is a good source of iron. Foods cooked in an iron skilled are absorbed better, increasing the bioavailability of iron.

In the US population, 7 percent of children aged one to five are iron deficient. These numbers are higher for Mexican Americans. In America, 10 per cent of women between 12 and 49 years of age are iron deficient. This number is 12 percent for Latinas and 16 percent for black women. These numbers are even higher in pregnant women. This is very concerning, since these deficiencies may affect the cognitive development of children.

Magnesium

Magnesium is another mineral that is important for the proper function of calcium and for the activity of vitamin D as it converts vitamin D into its active form. Magnesium is involved in the metabolism of carbohydrates and fats and the production of DNA, RNA, and many proteins. This mineral is involved in nerve and muscle activity and helps maintain the normal heart rhythm. Magnesium is necessary for the synthesis of glutathione, which is one of the most important antioxidants. It also helps to lower blood pressure by relaxing the blood vessels. Using magnesium as a supplement in the treatment of hypertension is a good idea. In pregnant women with preeclampsia, magnesium helps to lower blood pressure, reducing the risks of seizures or death of the mother. Magnesium prevents sudden cardiac death, which is responsible for more than fifty percent of cardiac deaths. Studies have shown that people with low magnesium levels (less than 1.77 mg/dL) have a higher risk of atrial fibrillation. A Japanese study showed that people with higher intake of magnesium have a lower risk of developing a stroke or heart failure.

Magnesium helps to maintain normal blood sugar levels, preventing diabetes. Studies have shown that increasing the intake of magnesium may lower the risk of diabetes by 22 percent. When blood sugar rises, magnesium is excreted in the urine. This causes a deficiency of magnesium in diabetics. Scientific studies suggest that using magnesium supplementation is protective and helps to decrease inflammation.

Magnesium increases enzyme activity that helps your body use vitamin D and regulates calcium. All enzymes that metabolize vitamin D require magnesium to work. As with vitamin D and K2, a magnesium deficiency is present in many people. If you are low in magnesium and take supplemental calcium, you may exacerbate the situation. If you take a calcium supplement, you should include magnesium, vitamin D, and K2. Magnesium helps to relax muscles, prevents cramps, and helps people to relax and sleep. Low levels of magnesium reduce serotonin levels, which leads to depression. People with anxiety and depression feel better with magnesium supplementation.

Magnesium has many benefits. For example, several studies show that it is superior to ibuprofen and naproxen in treating migraines. Magnesium with vitamin B6 helps to reduce menstrual cramps, anxiety, and irritability. It also decreases breast tenderness, menstrual weight gain, and pain. Taking magnesium at night helps to reduce muscle cramps, promoting a good restful sleep. Magnesium helps to elevate levels of good HDL or good cholesterol. IV magnesium is very helpful for patients with severe asthma that does not respond to other medications. I usually recommend magnesium to people with insomnia and fibromyalgia.

Dietary sources of magnesium include many vegetables, like spinach, black beans, pumpkin seeds, almonds, cashews, peanut butter, avocados, wheat bread, brown rice, yogurt, salmon, milk, dark chocolate, and sea vegetables. Taking too much calcium and salt causes loss of magnesium and low levels of magnesium. Women on oral contraceptives who have low levels of magnesium are at risk of developing blood clots and strokes. Women who complain of headaches while taking contraceptives should take magnesium supplements.

As for supplements, magnesium citrate and magnesium threonate are among the best. An optimal dose of magnesium is 400 mg a day. Too much magnesium citrate can cause diarrhea. In fact, magnesium citrate is used to treat constipation. It is available in bottles that look like a soda. Half of the bottle is sometimes enough to relieve constipation since it is a good laxative. Magnesium gels and lotions help to relax muscles and reduce muscle cramps. Since magnesium can be absorbed through the skin to some degree, bathing with Epsom salts (magnesium sulfate) helps to relax muscles. There are many commercial preparations of calcium, magnesium, and vitamin D in liquid form that are very useful in creating a good balance of these important minerals and assisting with many functions in the body.

Magnesium helps to increase the production of melatonin. Taking magnesium at night with foods rich in melatonin helps to restore normal circadian rhythms. Foods rich in melatonin include almonds, spinach, avocados, pineapples, oranges, and bananas. You can prepare a salad using all these foods with salmon every night to help you sleep better. My "Nice Sleep Salad" is a way to help those with sleeping problems to increase their melatonin levels. See Appendix F. Melatonin is a hormone that decreases by 14 percent every decade. It is no wonder that we may have difficulties in sleeping as we age!

Zinc and boron

Zinc and boron are other important cofactors that interact with vitamin D. Zinc deficiency has also been identified as a contributing factor to Alzheimer's disease. Zinc helps to strengthen the immune system, heal wounds, improve skin rashes and problems, decrease inflammation of the prostate, and improve the sense of smell and taste. Zinc is involved in the normal growth and development of organs and tissues. It is present in shellfish, red meat, poultry, beans, nuts, and whole grains. The body does not store zinc, and deficiencies are common in people with inflammation, arthritis, diabetes, and intestinal absorption problems. Pregnant women with zinc deficiencies may have premature babies, who in turn may have abnormal growth and development. Zinc is involved in the expression of many genes and is present in the cell nucleus to repair defective DNA, replication, and transcription. Men need a higher daily requirement of zinc because it is used in the production of testosterone. Zinc concentration is high in the prostate gland, testes, and sperm. When men are deficient in zinc, they suffer low testosterone and infertility.

Zinc is important to maintain a strong immune system because it activates T lymphocytes responsible for destroying cells infected with viruses and bacteria or cells that have become cancerous. Other white cells like macrophages, neutrophils, and killer cells use zinc to increase their defensive role against infection. When a person has a cold, it is better to use zinc instead of vitamin C. Zinc lozenges reduce the severity of a cold if taken within twenty-four hours after the onset of symptoms.

Zinc is involved in the production of collagen and healing of wounds. Zinc activates collagenase, an enzyme involved in the production of collagen. As people age or the skin develops wrinkles, collagen is lost in the dermis. Taking zinc helps to activate collagenase to keep producing collagen to restore the structure of the dermis and decrease the effects of aging. Zinc is also involved in the mineralization of bones and makes them stronger and less likely to break.

Zinc is a structural component of many antioxidants that help to prevent damage by free radicals through a process of oxidative stress. Zinc is present in superoxide dismutase, the most powerful antioxidant, which is also a powerful anti-inflammatory. When zinc levels are low, the synthesis of powerful antioxidant enzymes decreases, and the level of oxidative stress increases, exposing the DNA to more damage. Because people with diabetes have higher levels of DNA damage, they may be more susceptible to cancer.

Zinc helps our vision when combined with vitamin A. It helps to produce a retinal-binding protein, which delivers vitamin A to the retina to improve night vision. When combined with antioxidants, zinc helps to prevent macular degeneration and blindness. Zinc protects red and inflamed gums and prevents canker sores. In 2012, a study published in the *Journal of Affective Disorders* suggested that zinc supplementation is beneficial in treating depression when combined with antidepressants.

Prolonged intake and higher doses of zinc might affect levels of copper.

Boron is a trace mineral found in many fruits and vegetables. It is important for bone health because it helps to prevent calcium loss. It also helps to increase the production of sex hormone and build muscles for athletic performance. A supplement of 3 mg a day is enough to maintain bone health. Best sources are apples, broccoli, and root vegetables.

The best advice and to make it simple is to take a multivitamin that contains all minerals once a day. I recommend different multivitamins in Appendix A. For specific deficiencies and problems of absorption from the gut, it's better to take the vitamins separately to address the deficiency. Children, pregnant women, vegetarians, and people who drink alcohol are at higher risk of developing mineral deficiencies. A good multivitamin helps to keep our bodies in balance, perfect equilibrium, and prevent deficiencies. Vegetarians need additional vitamin B12. Diabetics need complex B vitamins and some minerals in higher dosages. Chromium picolinate, 500 mg, a day may help to increase insulin sensitivity, lower triglycerides, and raise good cholesterol (HDL).

People taking cholesterol-lowering drugs benefit by taking CoQ10 and vitamin K2 to prevent plaque formation in the coronary arteries.

Diet and the Coming Longevity Revolution

What can you do to keep your body in balance?

Managing your diet and adding proper minerals and supplements will help you to join the longevity revolution. Eating healthy foods and keeping you weight in check require information. You also need lots of willpower and discipline to keep your body functioning at optimal levels. In this book, I have already given you information about healthy diets, minerals, and supplements to help you stay healthy and keep your body in balance. Our bodies are like vehicles. If they are maintained well, they will give us more years of good use. As we age, most cells begin to slow down and produce fewer hormones. Sometimes, we are unaware of these changes, and the deficiency continues. When the levels of a hormone produced by the cells drops significantly, we begin to feel weak or become ill. My advice is to check with your doctor and have the levels of most hormones checked for deficiencies. You can do the same for micronutrients like iron, magnesium, vitamin D, folic acid, and vitamin B12, among others.

If you do not pay attention to the changes taking place in your body, many cells eventually will stop functioning and die. If more cells begin to fail and are unattended, many organs and systems also will begin to fail. These failures, in turn, cause changes in your skin, bones, muscles, and brain. At this point, you may begin to experience weight gain or loss, hot flashes, hair loss, increased pain, anxiety, weakness, fatigue, decreased libido, and depression. Your sleep may be disrupted as well, and your overall feeling of health will be diminished. Your short-term memory and intellectual activities may begin to deteriorate gradually as well. The good news is that all these changes can be reversed if they are diagnosed in time and treated properly. You just have to make a choice and decide. Procrastination and inaction are also killers. You must decide to bring your body in balance to restore and maintain the proper equilibrium within your cells and bring your hormone functions, organs, and systems back to perfect balance throughout your life span.

Nutritional and hormonal assessment

With our current knowledge, we can assess our nutritional status and health. A doctor qualified to provide nutritional and hormonal assessment could undertake a comprehensive analysis of all micronutrients, including all vitamins, essential fatty acids (omega-3, -6, and -9), antioxidants, hormones, and all other chemistries to understand serum levels and function. You should start with your family doctor or internist to request all these tests. He may want to refer you to a specialist if your problem is due to hormone imbalances. Specialists in endocrinology evaluate all types of hormonal problems. Some doctors subspecialize in complementary and alternative medicine. You can check the board of specialties and the listings in your local area for these specialists. Some other diagnostic tests to assess other conditions may require targeted testing. They may include testing to assess metabolic functions, cardiovascular problems, arthritis and connective tissue disorders, and genetic disorders. You may want a telomere assessment to determine biological age and life expectancy. These assessments have important clinical applications to rebalance deficiencies and correct potential or existing problems. Check the resource section of this book and resources for additional information.

Taking a proactive approach is the best way to prevent deficits before they become symptomatic. Today, specialized laboratories offer methods to assess nutrients at the intracellular level for a better understanding of how these micronutrients are affecting specific cells and our overall systems.

It is also possible to assess lymphocyte function, lymphocyte growth, mitogenic division, and genetic structure through DNA testing as well as do telomere testing to assess biological age and longevity. Genomic testing helps to prevent premature suffering and death from cancer or other chronic illnesses. BRCA1 and BRCA2 genetic testing detect genes that predispose women to breast or ovarian cancer. By acting before cancer develops, women can survive and live long normal lives. Today, many insurance companies pay for bilateral mastectomies and reconstruction if these genes are present. Knowledge of the presence of these two genes is important before a woman decides about hormone replacement therapy.

How nutritional deficiencies affect the telomeres

Certain diets will cause the telomeres to become shorter over time, shortening life span. A diet that is rich in refined sugar, sucrose, fructose, and syrups is one. Inflammatory diets, or diets which increase oxidative stress and include red meats, processed meats, white bread, sodas, saturated fats, omega-6 polyunsaturated fats, heavy alcohol consumption, and excessive iron supplements also shorten telomeres. These diets may be shortening your life and health span, as well.

As mentioned in the introduction, Drs. Blackburn and Epel have discovered how the telomeres shorten with each cell division to determine how fast the cells age and when they die. What is extraordinary is to know what causes the shortening and what helps to lengthen them. Aging in our modern age is not necessarily a slippery slope toward infirmity and decay. We all are going to get older, but how we do that depends on our cellular health. In their work, these two remarkable researchers have found new meaning to the interaction and relationship between the human mind and the body. What surprised them was the fact that telomeres do not simply carry out commands issued by our genetic code. They appear to absorb the instructions we give to them as well. The way a person lives, in effect, can tell the telomeres to accelerate the aging process. However, the opposite is true as well. A healthy lifestyle and the foods we eat can determine how long we will live. All these factors can prevent premature aging at the cellular level. From their research, we can conclude that the keys for a healthy longevity must foster healthy cell renewal (Blackburn 2015).

Our cells divide during a life span a limited number of times. Some age earlier than others do. This explains why joints begin to degenerate in some people earlier than any other organs. The biologist Leonard Hayflick discovered the so-called "Hayflick limit." This is the maximum limit a cell can divide before it dies. Before they reach this stage, the cells become sluggish or senescent. In other words, they become senile. In our bodies, all cells—including stem cells—have telomeres to keep our bodies healthy. They have an enzyme called telomerase. As long as there is enough telomerase, the cells will continue to divide and remain healthy. When the cells become senile, it's more than likely that they will not produce enough telomerase. They cannot do their jobs like they used to and die. If these cells had been responsible for keeping our immune systems strong before becoming senile, they will no longer protect us. If a virus or bacterium attacks, we may become susceptible to serious infections or cancer. Our aging cells cannot defend our bodies anymore; they are dying and tired. As the telomeres shorten, the cells will die soon as well. This winding down happens as we enter our seventies and eighties. This is happening because our cells are no longer dividing and have reached their limit of division and existence. This is the Hayflick limit.

The good news is that we can do something to experience good health and have a healthier life span beyond those years. All is within our reach if we can lengthen our telomeres by a proper diet and behaviors. Preventing premature chronological aging and moving into a younger biological age is possible. This is what matters—moving from the fast lane of chronological age into the slower and healthier lane of biological age. These extraordinary findings explain why reversing aging is possible. As we suggested previously, in the near future, we may be able to find centenarians who look twenty or thirty or more years younger than their chronological age. That is why biological age is what matters.

The discovery of how foods interact to lengthen the telomeres or how free radicals can cause cancer by damaging our DNA is evolving. Cancer of the colon has been associated with the intake of overcooked red meat (Sesink et al. 1999). This happens because the mucosa of the colon is overwhelmed by the amount of carcinogens and free radicals after one meal. The same may happen with diets rich in nitrites. Bacon, salami, bologna, and many other processed meats are rich in nitrites and many other free radicals that can damage the DNA. Every day, we learn more about how many chemicals or free radicals act to damage our DNA. We have to recognize that free radicals constantly bombard us.

To prevent damage of the cells, genetic mutations, and shortening of the telomeres, a diet with a large amount and variety of antioxidants helps to provide an oxidative defense to reduce the damage done by free radicals and oxidative stress, which shortens the telomeres or damages the nuclear DNA. A basic diet made of fresh vegetables, fruits, fiber, omega-3s, and fresh fish helps to maintain the telomeres longer. To protect the damage done by free radicals, I have listed foods that help to prevent DNA damage. My DRESS-SS prescription of diet, rest, exercise, sleeping properly, and stress management (plus sexuality and spirituality) provides the keys for a healthier lifestyle and longevity. This book is the bridge that will take you to the longevity world. It is your guide to build such structure through a lifestyle of wellness.

To assess the length of the telomeres, there are specific tests that can be correlated with diet and nutritional deficiencies. Correcting these nutritional deficiencies and changing eating habits can help to increase the length of the telomeres, prolong life, and prevent mutations. For a more effective defense, I also recommend decreasing caloric intake. There is no need to eat three times a day or have full meals every night. Eating before going to bed is also not a good idea because midnight binge eating will make you gain weight, which will affect the way your liver processes sugar while you sleep. Follow my fast-keto diet to maintain control of your weight and decrease the harmful effects of free radicals, lurking around and damaging your DNA and mitochondria.

Can we reverse aging with a healthy diet?

The answer to this question is a definite yes. Living longer and reversing aging requires a well-balanced diet. This is within our reach.

For a greater lifestyle of wellness and longer life spans, we should start early, as infants and during childhood, with a diet rich in micronutrients, healthy proteins, and good fats and carbohydrates. As a baseline, a healthy diet shouldn't have more than 30 grams of carbohydrates. Some may consider this amount too low, but it is a safer number than the one in the dietary guidelines—about twice this amount. A lower-carb diet will provide caloric restriction and less production of free radicals responsible for the damage to DNA and mitochondria. Athletes and persons involved in heavy activities that require higher levels of exercise and muscular activity require much higher levels of carbohydrates for optimal performance. However, they are not exempt of the higher production of free radicals that cause so much havoc and damage to DNA and mitochondria. To counter the effects of increased oxidative stress and inflammation due to heavy exercise, they must consume plenty of antioxidants to diminish the potential damage done to their cells and DNA.

Maintaining a normal BMI (normal body mass index is 18.5 to 24.9), in which weight is proportional to height, is a way to track ideal weight and excessive fat stored in our bodies.

The other effective way to maintain a normal BMI is to learn to utilize fat instead of carbohydrates as fuel. Earlier in this chapter, I recommended my fast-keto diet as a way to reduce caloric intake and use fat as fuel. Practicing intermittent fasting in the twenty-four-hour cycle helps to maintain normal weight and store more fat. My wife and I have been practicing this technique for years to keep our weight in check. You should also avoid inflammatory diets that trigger an inflammatory response in the body. Foods rich in fructose, refined sugars, lectins, and wheat germ agglutinins (WGA) may compromise the gut, encouraging autoimmune diseases, allergies, and leaky gut. Inflammation activates the NLRP3 gene, which triggers the production of cryopyrin, a protein that causes the inflammatory response that activates white cells to attack tissues and organs. A healthy microbiome made of good bacteria or probiotics prevents such attacks and damage to arteries, gut, and other tissues. Zinc, resveratrol, flavonoids, antioxidants, and drugs like metformin help to suppress inflammation.

Gut microbiome balance for a healthier lifestyle

There is another world inside of our gut full of trillions of microorganisms working for us to help to keep our bodies healthy and in balance. This ecosystem of microorganisms is a forgotten garden of life. We have evolved, assisted by this ecosystem to develop a strong immune system and transform many nutrients in substances that would help us to enjoy better health. When we treat this ecosystem poorly or destroy it with antibiotics or bad microorganisms and bad diets, this ecosystem is compromised, and we get sick. Balance and biodiversity in this ecosystem creates health and improves longevity. An imbalance and reduced biodiversity of this ecosystem creates illness (Mullin 2015, 5).

An imbalance of this ecosystem usually leads to weight gain and makes a person susceptible to many diseases.

The microbial flora has about 100 trillion microorganisms. They outnumber our human cells by a factor of ten to one. We have more bacterial organisms with their own DNA in the gut than we have human cells and DNA. It is clear that this huge universe of microorganisms has an impact on our health. The Human Microbiome Project has identified about a thousand species of microbes. There are different ecosystems that need to be analyzed. Our relationship with this ecosystem is symbiotic. We provide food to these microorganisms, and they help us in different ways. They help us to break down complex carbs and produce vitamins and nutrients like vitamin K, B12, niacin, pyridoxine, and many others. They also produce short-chain fatty acids and peptides important in fighting inflammation, regulate immunity, and protect us against cancer and many other diseases. These microfloras are our first line of defense against foreign microorganisms. They support detoxification and affect brain function, appetite, behavior, and mood. They also have a profound effect on our weight, health, and quality of life. A balanced system contributes to optimal weight and health. An imbalanced system leads to type 2 diabetes, irritable bowel syndrome (IBS), cardiovascular disease, allergies, and many other illnesses.

Eating too much sugar and fat and processed foods diminishes the biodiversity of microorganisms in the gut. This may lead to weight gain and obesity. Overuse of antibiotics has a detrimental effect in the intestinal microbiome because they kill billions of the microorganisms necessary to keep balance of this ecosystem and a good immune system. The lack of many of these good microorganisms may lead to problems in digesting many foods, resulting in diarrhea and loss of vital nutrients. The antibiotic threat is compounded by the use of antibiotics to feed chickens and cattle. This factor may be responsible for the increased rates of obesity in America due to an imbalanced microbiome.

There are good bacteria that help maintain a good balance and biodiversity in the gut. *Bifidobacterium breve* and *bifidum,* which enhance remission of IBS, are some of these. Some strains of lactobacillus are also very helpful. Others are very bad and may cause illness even in small quantities. *Salmonella* and *Shigella* are some of them. Most of the microorganisms live in the large intestine, but some are located in the small intestine. When too many bacteria move to the small intestine, they create a problem known as small intestine bacteria overgrowth (SIBO). Some of SIBO's symptoms are gas, bloating, flatulence after meals, loose stools, constipation, abdominal distention, and pain. Patients with chronic pain and fibromyalgia have SIBO symptoms. When SIBO is resolved, the symptoms improve and go away. People with SIBO symptoms gain weight. When SIBO is resolved, they lose weight. SIBO weakens the integrity of the intestinal lining, permitting bacterial toxins to escape and damage the liver. Changing to a healthy diet will make many of the symptoms of SIBO go away because that helps to eliminate the bad bacteria in favor of the good, for better balance. To enjoy a healthy lifestyle, you should have a healthy diet and microbiome to prevent SIBO.

Gerard Mullin, MD, in his book *Gut Balance Revolution*, recommends a program based on the three Rs to lose weight and restore you microbiome to balance.

The three Rs stand for reboot, rebalance, and renew. The reboot phase is when you "till the earth" to prepare the garden. You eliminate processed carbs and starch foods that cause all the SIBO symptoms. You start fat-burning superfoods like blueberries, green tea, and chili peppers. Rebalance is when you seed and fertilize you inner garden in your gut to restore ecological harmony. In this phase, you use more good fiber like artichokes; oat bran; and fermented foods like sauerkraut, kimchi, yogurt, kefir, and miso. In the renew phase, you keep your friendly flora happy to enjoy a healthy lifestyle. In this phase, you introduce more healthy foods; limit sugars; and eat healthy fibers, healthy fats, and healthy proteins.

Can we live longer if our bodies are in balance?

Yes! This is a goal. We can adjust and make changes to live longer and healthier. We have been living longer century after century and will continue to do so for centuries more. Many physicians and scientists believe that we can double our life spans or health spans within the next fifty years, if we keep our telomeres longer, keep our bodies in balance, and strive for optimal health. A revolution to stay younger and live longer has begun. We are not limited to living 100 to 120 years. We can expand the limits of our life spans with better lifestyles and nutrition. This is the purpose of this book. We are going to see millions of centenarians who look thirty to forty years younger in the next generation. My wife and I are a testament to this assertion. Keeping our bodies healthier decreases health care costs for the individual, the family, and the nation. As a physician, I predict there will be many changes in our bodies in the next century that will make us look younger and live longer. I believe we can improve our biological age if we have the determination to do something about it.

People will be amazed when our chronological age becomes less important and our biological age becomes the new reality that matters. This will not happen unless you make a choice and decide to be healthier and live longer. My DRESS-SS prescription is your password to this new reality and the key to enter this new world. You should start now and take the lead to undertake a more careful assessment of your nutritional and hormonal deficiencies, as well as your telomeres and telomerase levels to prevent early aging and subsequent organ and function decline. Applying my DRESS-SS formula will help you bring your body in balance and restore perfect equilibrium. You will be rewarded with better health and a younger look.

We should remember that we are part of the equilibrium in the universe. What has been happening to our planet for billions of years has affected us. Our lack of knowledge, ignorance, and neglect is what has caused our bodies at the cellular level to lose the internal balance necessary to prevent illness, premature aging, and death. By providing the proper nutrients and antioxidants to our cells, balancing our hormones as they change overtime, avoiding toxic nutrients that harm our bodies, controlling stress, enjoying deep and refreshing sleep every night, resting and taking frequent breaks, meditating, and enjoying a spiritual life, we can stop premature aging and improve our health. By following these practices, we can expect to look younger and healthier as we get older, rather than just accepting a long life with failing health.

The journey to stop cancer, arthritis, heart disease, and many other illnesses continues every day. Many cures are at hand and not far away. Very soon, we will be able to conquer many of the problems that shorten our lives and health spans. My DRESS-SS prescription is my best advice to you and your family. My prescription is the beginning of a better life and a healthy longevity. You should view life as a marathon, where you are expected to reach the goal line in the best possible shape. I want you to think that way. I am sure you want to age gracefully and enjoy life, walking unassisted and breathing on your own without the aid of an oxygen tank when you reach the goal line. I believe most of us want to reach old age healthier and looking many years younger than our peers of the same chronological age. There is no reason you can't achieve these goals. This is possible today. You just have to look at me and my wife. Please see our pictures in this book and judge by yourselves. Most importantly, read this book and jump to make a change for the better.

Once you develop the awareness of what is possible, you have to commit to follow my prescription to guide you to this new world of wellness, healthier longevity, and happiness, where you will make good choices. You should believe in yourself and make this reality possible. You also need to educate yourself and read more about what is best for you to stay healthy and then act. Thinking but failing to act is not an option. Procrastinating is not a solution. Life is too short to waste a moment or an opportunity to improve you health and longevity. You need discipline and determination to make this change possible. Your well-being and a happier, healthy longevity is your responsibility and is in your hands. *Living Longer and Reversing Aging* is a guide to help you to reach your ultimate goal for optimal health and happiness. It does not matter how old you are; it's never too late or too early to begin to assess your health, to make changes, and to act. I encourage you to start today. Keep this book with you all the time. Get the digital version to check anything you want when you have a break, when buying groceries, or when enjoying free time. This book has a great deal of information to make you happier and help you live longer. Share this information with your friends and family. Invite them to this new world of healthier longevity. Let them know there is a book to help them cross the bridge and reach their destination. If you are a couple, make this book an essential guide to maintain a healthier lifestyle together. Remember, happiness is the ultimate goal. I want you to use this book to enhance your health and level of happiness. If you can add a few more years to your life and live healthier, delay aging, and be happier, you should feel rewarded. The younger you start to assess changes and live a healthier lifestyle, the greater the reward.

As we age, we also grow in wisdom, and this wisdom will become a gift to humankind and the younger generations. As we age, we mature and grow spiritually as well. This mature spirituality is a blessing for you, your loved ones, your friends, and humanity. I have no doubt that boomers who are living longer will have a significant influence on how we will live in the future. As millions of people pay more attention to their health, more knowledge and changes for the better will come their way. Currently, boomers contribute more than $7 trillion to the economy, and in fifteen more years, the impact of their contributions will surpass $20 trillion. Prolonging age and years of gainful activity and wisdom may become a bonanza for families; companies; the national economy; teaching institutions engaged in research, science, and medicine; and better health care for many nations. Knowledge, wisdom, and experience that remain for many decades are a gift to humanity. A healthy longevity will prevent such loss.

Start this longevity revolution today. Begin by being aware of how to improve your health and how to correct deficiencies. Remember that, by keeping your body healthy through positive actions, you will also improve your mind and spirit. Keeping your body healthy at the cellular level is an important concept that will help keep your organ functions in check for a perfect balance and help you achieve good health, stay younger, and live longer. Elite athletes, Olympic men and women, should use this book and my prescription to achieve strength, optimal health, and endurance to be successful in any competitive sport. The more your mind and body are in perfect equilibrium, the greater your success.

DRESS-SS is my prescription to live a healthier long life and reverse aging. I also call this prescription a code or formula for a better life or a healthier lifestyle. This is your foundation for healthy and joyful living. Although diet is very important, diet is not enough. You need to build on this foundation by introducing rest, exercise, healthy sleep, and stress management into your daily routine. All these actions create the basic structure to cross the bridge that will lead you to a healthy, happy, satisfied lifestyle of wellness.

CHAPTER 3
R is for Rest

Everybody deserves a break

We all need to take a break during our waking hours. When life is too busy, it is difficult to be on top of everything. The busier we are, the greater our level of stress. Life is a marathon for many people. We cannot run marathons every day without a break or rest. Breaks are important to unwind and recover our concentration, regain energy, and continue to move on to bring balance to our lives. Rest is the easiest way to find a way to maintain your health and sanity. It is important to take breaks during the day, even if they are short. Sleep, which is an important form of rest, will be discussed in another chapter. Taking vacations once or twice a year to unwind helps us to find and restore balance before returning to work or school. Breaks and vacations give us more energy and motivation. During this time, our levels of adrenaline and cortisol drop to give us a feeling of relaxation.

If you work, attend school, or are involved in an activity that demands many hours of your life each day, you should take breaks to rest you body and mind. A short break of five to ten minutes throughout the day helps you collect your thoughts and reduce stress. A short five-minute walk helps to improve mood, boost energy, reduce fatigue, and improve creativity and concentration. This is a good habit to practice.

Calling or texting is not a way of getting the rest that your mind and body needs. To enjoy the benefits of a break, you should turn off your phone or leave it in the car or office for a few minutes. The same should happen at dinnertime. You should engage your spouse, friends, family, and children during meals. It is a bad habit to use your phone while enjoying a meal with them. Socialization and the exchange of ideas and emotions stimulate the mind and contribute to keeping in contact with our loved ones. Social breaks or spending time with others reduces stress and improves mood. When your mind is always wondering about the next call or message, you are not taking a break. There will be always time for another call or to text a message or check your emails.

If you are under a great deal of stress, you especially need to find time for more breaks each day. Most people who suffer from excessive stress never take time to meditate and rewind. The brain waves continue at such a rapid pace that the brain interprets this state as a fight-or-flight reaction. Stress doesn't allow your body to decrease the release of adrenaline and cortisone. Some people may feel anxious or develop panic attacks and don't understand what is happening to them. Rather than taking a tranquilizer, it is much better to take a break, rest your mind to collect your thoughts, and relax. You need to review your lifestyle and make a list of the tasks or activities that are important every day and prioritize them if you are always in a hurry or feel too much stress.

For more information on dealing with stress, I want you to read chapter 5, which deals with stress. Good actions that bring more pleasure and happiness should be at the top of your list. Discard what is not important or brings you too much stress or unhappiness. Use a calendar or schedule to organize your time and prioritize what is important. Do not spend time on trivial matters that waste time. Learn to say *no* to your friends and family by declining some invitations politely. Limit your commitments and meetings to important matters to reduce your stress, and you will find more time to take breaks and rest your mind and body.

Remember that there are only twenty-four hours in the day, and at least eight should be reserved for sleep if you want to live a healthy lifestyle. Skimping on sleep is a bad strategy. When you fail to sleep enough hours, you will feel tired the following day. Prolonged sleep deprivation will affect your health and shorten your life span. I will address the importance of good refreshing sleep in chapter "S is for Sleep."

When making a list to organize your time and finding time for more breaks, limit your main actions to a few things. Making a long list is overwhelming. Do not waste energy on petty matters. Be positive and approach everything with an open mind. When I have several bills to pay or matters to address, I make a list the night before. This helps me sleep better and decreases the brain activity before going to bed. Many people have a hard time unwinding and going to sleep at night because the brain continues with the beta rhythm as if they are awake. People with excessive stress, worries, anxiety, or lingering thoughts have a hard time falling asleep. Learning to take breaks to unwind during the day helps you to prepare to unwind at night before going to sleep. Rest is like a medicine that would help you bring balance to your mind.

My prescription is based on a commitment to balance your body and emotional state for ultimate happiness. I included rest as part of my prescription because many of my patients complain of a great deal of stress and difficulties sleeping at night. The problem all of them have is a lack of time to collect their thoughts and relax. A relaxing break gives your body and mind time to pause and boost your energy and enthusiasm. I have been practicing short breaks and relaxation for years, and it works. My blood pressure is ten points below the normal and very rarely is five points above the normal. I learned to control my emotions while I worked in the emergency room during my medical training. I knew that I had to remain cool to be able to help a person in pain with a broken arm or a leg or someone with great deal of pain. It takes practice, and I want you to take more frequent short breaks to learn to relax, boost your energy, and improve your mental capacity for a balanced and happier well-being. Failure to take breaks and unwind eventually will damage your health. The constant high levels of adrenaline and cortisol are unhealthy.

While you rest or take a break, you should learn to meditate and think what makes you happy. Remember our goal in life is to be happy and you should do everything possible to enjoy this feeling all the time. Happiness is a state of peace and ongoing life satisfaction. It conveys a deep feeling of connection, with the mind and spirit allowing us to move ahead and enjoy human connections and everything we do that fulfills our every daily lives. Happiness starts with our thoughts and is something we create for ourselves. It is a feeling of joy, wellness, satisfaction, and gratitude that transcends any material possessions or attending a telephone all the time. You do not have to be rich or have money to feel great happiness. Happiness is intangible, abundant, and free. You can get as much happiness as you want. It all depends on you. Being positive and having a positive attitude and purpose in life helps to enhance this powerful feeling. Practicing gratitude and compassion deepens your happiness. Your thoughts guide your level of happiness. You must take the time to rest, think about the things that make you happy, and enjoy this feeling while in the moment. Transport yourself to the past and think about something that made you happy, enjoy the memory and the feeling, bring this good memory to the present, and project it to the future. This is an exercise that will help you to keep good memories active, where you can go anytime you feel under stress. Practicing this form of "meditation" several times a day is medicine to the soul.

Many doctors neglect to offer or give their patients this kind of advice, so I am giving it to you. It is free and works anywhere in the world. Try it and experience it. Any moment of happiness is precious and rewarding. Moreover, if practiced every day, it brings healing beyond your imagination. Enjoy the present and every moment. Remember, it is not how much money you have or make or what possessions you have that give you this feeling of happiness; it is your state of mind and your thoughts that make you feel happy. To increase your level of happiness, look for friends who are happy, kind, and compassionate. Friends who are positive and happy rub off on us. Avoid, as much as possible, people who are negative, have negative attitudes, or are sad all the time. They do not bring happiness. You express a happy attitude by your work, actions, and words. People will notice that you are a happy person wherever you are. Happiness will follow you everywhere if you take breaks from the daily routine.

Turn the break into something positive and uplifting. Meditate and convey your feelings through positive words, facial expressions, actions, tone of voice, moods, and posture. Transmit happiness through written words, messages, pictures, acts of kindness, and compassion. If you have a partner, you can make a commitment to find happiness in the relationship every day if both take the time to empathize with each other's feelings and express love. Some married men say, "A happy wife is a happy life." This is true. A man who takes time to do what makes his wife happy most likely is a happy man. If he shows kindness, empathy, compassion, and love for her, she will love him in return. The same can be applied to partners or family members living with you. Learning to deflect conflict and negative feelings by approaching events and actions with an open and positive mind shows love and kindness.

My wife and I practice this approach. I actually feel happy when my wife is happy, and she reciprocates. This approach to our daily life and decisions reduces stress and enhances our happiness. Happiness is superior to conflict, so never sacrifice happiness for conflict, anger, jealousy, or negative feelings.

Happiness is too precious to compromise over petty matters or arguments. If there is conflict, think about what is important to you and your partner before you sacrifice your level of happiness. Take a break to remove the negative element.

You should also take breaks and go for a walk with your partner or friend. Talking without being judgmental helps to enhance the relationship and level of happiness. A loving call to your partner could be a form of a resting break. Always project love and avoid making calls to project anger and hate. This is not helpful. Love and happiness is more valuable and healing than anger, jealousy, or hate. My prescription is based on your desire to pursue love and happiness in life.

You can meditate for a few minutes to enjoy the moment and relax the mind every day. For those with too much stress and anxiety, I recommend another form of meditation called "mindfulness meditation." Mindfulness meditation is a good way to take a break from your daily activities. I explain this form of meditation in more detail in the chapter 5, which addresses stress and stress management. It is important to set aside time to meditate when you face conflict or an unexpected event. Wait a few seconds before responding and uttering a hateful word or remark in response to hateful questions loaded with negative words from someone who wants to hurt your feelings.

It is also wise to take a break to think before you enter into a potentially stressful situation, just as you would before signing a financial document or a contract that may cause legal problems down the road. Taking time to think and collect your thoughts is a good practice that helps reduce stress. Whenever you are in doubt about how to proceed with an important decision, ask yourself whether this decision will make you happy or not. Will this decision or action hurt you or your family in any way? Will your words hurt or carry negative feelings or hurt someone else with serious consequences? If the answer is *yes*, you should wait longer and take time to think until you are ready with your answer. It is not a good idea to take risks when you are under pressure or duress. You may regret your decisions later since a bad decision may cause more stress and ultimately decrease your happiness. Taking a break to rest is the wise solution when in doubt.

Rest is not limited to everyday decisions. Planning for leisure time is important to keep a healthy mind and body. Our beta brain waves are running at full speed during the day. The greater the pressure, the greater the stress we experience. Stress raises the levels of cortisol and adrenaline to prepare you for a "fight-or-flight" decision. Constant high levels of these substances and other neurotransmitters eventually take a toll on your physical and mental health. Rest is essential for good health. For centuries, Spaniards have taken naps to feel refreshed during the day. Winston Churchill used to take naps to be able to work late at night. He said he was able to make better decisions after taking a nap. He was correct. Brain waves slow down when we sleep. When we go into deep sleep, the brain has time to refresh and repair any damage. Unfortunately, it is hard in our modern and stressful world to take naps as the Spaniards or Churchill did to stay calm, relieve their stress, and maintain their sanity.

It is wise to take a lunch break and a walk to unwind after working all morning. This is the time to practice mindfulness meditation, which I explain in more detail chapter 5, which talks about stress management. Companies should allow workers to have at least a one-hour break for lunch and rest to keep their employees healthier, happier, and more productive. Lunchtime or a break from work is a time to nourish the body and soul. It allows for a time to meditate for a few minutes to unwind the mind and reduce stress. After a refreshing lunch break, you will be more productive. A person who takes breaks and meditates feels less stress and is ready to take more assignments or continue a demanding task.

I caution you not to use this time for more argument or controversy or unnecessary phone calls. This is a time to diminish stress, live in the present, feel calm, and bring your body and soul to a moment of peace. You deserve to take this time to rest and find peace. You are entitled to be happy, and these few minutes of rest are to be enjoyed so that you can take a break from the state of "autopilot" in which so many people are living today. Do not make a call to anyone if you expect an angry response. Do not destroy the moment of peace you are enjoying. It is never a good idea to sacrifice happiness and peace for conflict and more stress. If the environment at work is too stressful, find more opportunities to take more short breaks during the day. A coffee break or a short walk to meditate and collect your thoughts is always beneficial to reduce your stress, think better, stay healthy, and live longer.

A healthy lifestyle in a twenty-four-hour cycle is not possible without deep and refreshing sleep. Working overtime or graveyard shifts carries significant stress. Prolonged work at night leads to physiological changes and serious deficiencies with deleterious effects that reduce your overall physical and emotional health and your happiness. People who suffer with insomnia or sleep deprivation do not produce enough growth hormone, which is necessary to repair our cell functions and organs. Our bodies produce this hormone at night during deep sleep. We can't change our physiological clocks that have been operating for millions of years in one week or a month. If you work overtime or graveyards, limit these shifts to no more than three days a week. Then, in your days off, take time to restore your normal cycle. Your mind and your body are precious, and they should be your concern. More overtime money in exchange for bad health is not a wise choice. Forty hours a week is more than enough for any working activity that demands concentration, constant physical activity, or a great deal of stress. However, just getting a good night's sleep is not always enough. Rest or breaks during the day are necessary to manage the stress most jobs demand, and the need is greater the greater the level of stress. My recommendation to people under a great deal of stress at work is to take more breaks, meditate, and enjoy the present. Relish every moment you are at peace during the day and sleep eight hours at night.

Remember, you are the guardian of your body and your mind, and it is your job to protect them. Your mind—through your thoughts—should assume control and protect your body from any harm. Rest is part of the plan to heal your body and repair the damage caused by stress if you want a longer, healthier life. Take vacations to unwind, reduce stress, and refresh your mind and body. Getting away from your daily routine and environment gives you time to catch up with your sleep and relationships.

Visiting family, friends, and loved ones gives perspective and purpose to your life. Humans have a great need to recall the past and rekindle close relationships with family and friends. Many individuals become anxious or depressed when time has passed and they have not seen aging parents or love ones for some time. Feeling their love again and expressing gratitude is stimulating and refreshing. Feeling their love and recharging your "love batteries" is a great way to regain joy and fulfillment in your life. Expressing your love and gratitude, followed by acts of kindness, helps you to repair the damage done to your bodies by the daily stress and excesses at work or at home.

Life is too short, and every moment counts in a pursuit of happiness. Enjoy every moment of peace and calm. Relaxing on a beach or enjoying a beautiful landscape brings a stimulating perspective to our lives. A week or two weeks of vacation may be sufficient to bring down the level of stress. Vacations twice a year should be the norm to achieve better balance. Get sufficient sleep and take frequent breaks or naps if possible. Meditate and take time to collect your thoughts, show gratitude, be kind and compassionate, and stay in the present. Practicing these simple actions will help you to rest your body and mind, reduce your stress, and allow you to experience more happiness.

CHAPTER 4

E is for Exercise

The importance of movement

Our bodies are made to move. Exercise is essential for the achievement of good health and healing. Exercise brings more blood flow to the brain, muscles, and tissues to stay healthy and promote healing. When we exercise, our hearts also get a workout, which improves circulation through the heart, brain, muscles, ligaments, joints, bones, skin, and organs.

When we sustain an injury to an arm or a leg that requires the immobilization of the joints in a cast or a brace, our muscles shrink or become atrophic, a condition called "atrophy of disuse." To recover, we need physical therapy to stretch the stiff joint and progressive resistive exercise to recover our strength once the brace or the cast is removed.

During my training in physical medicine and rehabilitation and my years of practice, which included treating many people with sports injuries, I had the opportunity to see patients with all types of orthopedic and neurological injuries. It is amazing how quickly muscles deteriorate and how rapidly we lose our strength. In the past, doctors had patients resting in bed for days or weeks and did not allow them to walk or exercise. When they were allowed to get out of bed, they felt dizzy and could not stand and walk. Today, when a person has an injury that limits walking or consciousness, doctors prescribe physical therapy to prevent atrophy and weakness. They also allow activity and movement as soon as possible to prevent deconditioning.

The same principle applies to your body when you become a "couch potato" or do not exercise. As the muscles become atrophic and weak, the heart also becomes weaker because it is out of shape and is not prepared to carry an increased load. This is common as we age. As we get older, our natural functions decline. Elderly people often remain in chairs or wheelchairs for hours a day. This leads to rapid deterioration of the brain and the muscular system. It is no surprise that they fall and break a hip or another bone. They are too weak to stand and walk. Eventually, they become bedridden and die prematurely from complications of a fracture or injury. All these complications can be prevented.

We must commit to exercise every day from fifteen to thirty minutes to stay fit. If we can exercise longer, it is even better. The more time you want to dedicate to exercise, the better. Adults who exercise at least three times a week have a 30 to 40 percent lower risk of developing dementia later in life than those who don't exercise.

Where do we get the energy to exercise?

When we are born, our cells grow fast and are full of energy. This energy comes from a specialized system in the mitochondria inside the cells. The cells need glucose, which is transported by insulin and delivered to the mitochondria to start the process of creating energy. When people develop resistance to transporting glucose inside the cells, blood sugar rises, and the cells do not have enough sugars entering the mitochondria to produce energy for all the vital functions. This disturbance causes a person to feel weak. This is common in prediabetics and those with type 2 diabetes.

Glucose, or blood sugar, is the fuel that produces energy to carry out all physiological functions and is essential to exercise. An adequate amount of carbohydrates is necessary for healthy cell function. In my experience, an excessive amount of sugar in the diet is the reason for insulin resistance and the cause of type 2 diabetes. The lack of a normal glucose metabolism affects how we feel, and it determines the strength we need to perform our daily activities and exercise. When blood sugar is low, we have hypoglycemia and feel very weak. When blood sugar is too high, we may feel dizzy and thirsty and develop acidosis, which can lead to a loss of consciousness.

A normal glucose metabolism is necessary for the healthy function of all cells, particularly our muscle and nerve cells, which use most of the glucose to provide energy to our bodies. Exercise helps to burn blood sugar and regulates type 2 diabetes. Diet and exercise are the best ways to treat type 2 diabetes without medications. That is why these two activities are part of our longevity code to live healthier and longer. I have many patients who had gastric bypasses to treat obesity and who were diabetics on insulin. Once they lost significant weight, most of them found they no longer required insulin.

When we consume a meal rich in carbohydrates, our pancreas produces insulin to lower and regulate the level of sugar circulating in the blood. Insulin is a hormone that helps to transport sugar inside the cells. Sugar is transported to the mitochondria, which is an energy powerhouse inside the cell.

Inside the mitochondria, sugar is metabolized into CO_2, water, and energy in the form of ATP and free radicals. This is how we get the energy to exercise. Athletes require high-carbohydrate diets since they need larger amounts of energy to accomplish their tasks. If the diet is deficient in carbohydrates, the athlete may feel weak, tired, and unable to complete the task. In diabetics, too much sugar or carbohydrates are harmful. Too much sugar makes their diabetes worse. Eating too much or consuming refined sugars makes people gain weight. Even after one heavy meal, a person can gain three or four pounds. If you continue to eat heavy meals, over time it becomes very difficult to lose weight due to accumulation of fat and water retention.

Losing weight helps prevent type 2 diabetes. Exercise helps burn the excess of blood sugar. For every kilogram we lose, we lower the risk of diabetes by 16 percent. Many studies estimate that a high percentage of cases of heart attacks are related to poor diets, too much stress, lack of exercise, and poor sleeping habits. My longevity prescription, when applied properly, will prevent premature aging and death. Balancing your carbohydrate intake will keep your body functions healthy. Overwhelming your cells and the mitochondria with too many sugars is destructive to your body. They do not need excessive energy sources, and the excess of free radicals may damage the mitochondria and the DNA and possibly cause cancer.

Cardio (aerobic) and strengthening (anaerobic) exercises or both?

There are different kinds of exercises. If you want to maintain cardiovascular endurance, you need cardio exercises. This kind of exercise is also known as aerobic exercise because it uses oxygen to meet exercise demands during aerobic metabolism. This is a form of light to moderate exercise and doesn't require heavy lifting. This can be accomplished by walking, running, bicycling, or swimming. Fifteen to twenty minutes of exercise is fine for anyone over sixty on a daily basis. Younger people should double this amount of cardio exercise. Walking on a treadmill or bicycling on a stationary bicycle works to fulfill this requirement. What is important is to raise your heart rate to about 70 percent of the predicted normal cardiac rate for the person's age. The formula to estimate the maximum cardiac rate is as follows: First, multiply your age by 70 percent (.7). Second, subtract this number from 208. For example, if your age is 30: $30 \times 7 = 21$; $208 - 21 = 187$. This is the maximum heart rate to exercise for a person aged thirty.

For more information about aerobic exercises, there are many videos on YouTube that explain the exercises. You can also find low- and high-impact exercise videos to design your exercise program. Many hospitals offer cardiac rehab programs in case of coronary artery disease to monitor your exercise program. Basically, the idea is not to build levels of lactate associated with muscle pain. People with coronary disease, however, must exercise with caution following the advice of a doctor based on a cardiac stress test.

Strength training is another form of exercise. If you want to increase muscle mass or improve muscle tone and strength, strengthening exercises meet the challenge. The exercises require some type of resistance. PRE, or progressive resistance exercise, utilizes weights, elastic strings, or special equipment found in a gym to accomplish this goal. Small weights at home can help to improve strength too. Anyone who is interested in living healthier and longer must exercise regularly. I recommend both cardio and strength training.

Exercise is something you can enjoy with others. One type of enjoyable exercise is dancing. My wife and I like dancing. It is a great exercise and helps a couple to function as a team. Dancing creates a mood of happiness and togetherness, which I do not find in any other sport. I recommend that people take dancing lessons to enjoy the music, the exercise, the positive feelings, and the joy when you dance. Dancing helps to improve balance, coordination, posture, heart function, muscle strength, bone density, and joint flexibility. Dancing creates a positive mood and a feeling of joy. Dancing sharpens the mind and helps you think faster. The social component helps you increase your competitive nature and improves your memory, attention, and concentration. As we age, we lose strength, speed, and coordination.

Dancing prevents this decline. Whether you are single or married, I encourage you to contact a dance center nearby and take lessons. Invite a friend to make your encounters more meaningful and exciting. Many places offer affordable classes in groups. You can also meet other people to dance with if you have no partner. Most teachers and students are usually very friendly. Many centers encourage people to dance with each other and socialize.

Men are often reluctant to dance; they do not know what they are missing. I didn't know how to dance until I was fifty. One day, my wife invited me to join a dance center to take lessons. After a few sessions, I was hooked. This was an enjoyable experience. We eventually went to national competitions for over ten years. We still dance socially, and the exercise helps us stay in great shape. Women love to dance and look beautiful when they go to dance. In a good marriage, dancing should be one of the couple's hobbies because it is a way to grow older and stay in great shape and feel happy.

Walking and bicycling outdoors is also an enjoyable form of getting aerobic exercise. A great exercise for those with arthritis or painful knees or feet is swimming. You can strengthen your arms and develop good cardiovascular endurance and expand your lungs when you swim. Many YWCA centers have heated swimming pools and offer exercise and dance classes.

My wife and I also exercise every day at home. We have a treadmill and barbells. Clara uses cuff weights to strengthen her leg muscles. Walking for ten minutes on the treadmill provides cardio exercise. We also exercise in place and stretch the lower back and leg muscles.

A person can design a personalized program depending on what area needs emphasis. Today, you can find many free programs on YouTube so that you can exercise at home. You also can find dancing lessons on You Tube if you don't have time to go to a dancing center.

How does exercise aid in recovery from an injury?

If you have sustained an injury to a muscle, a ligament, or a joint, the ligament or the muscle requires stretching due to prolonged immobilization or contracture. A therapist can provide passive range of motion exercises if the joint is very stiff or there is a muscle contracture. If you can move the joint, the therapist can provide active range of motion exercises, followed by progressive resistive exercises to improve strength. We use these terms in rehabilitation. A person can recover from an injury and recover strength gradually until reaching the maximum level of functioning. You should not hurry the process. Rehab may take weeks or months of intensive physical therapy to get the desired results. Ligaments and muscles are elastic, and they recover with exercise.

Low back pain is a common complaint. I frequently see people with this problem in my practice. It is very common in people who are sedentary and spend hours sitting at work or at home. Truck drivers, secretaries, and people with sedentary lifestyles suffer from this problem quite often. The reason for this pain is mechanical, resulting from tight muscles that have shortened due to inactivity. When the hamstrings and hip muscles become too tight, they pull the lumbar spine and increase the normal lumbar curvature of the spine, a condition known as lordosis. This in turn causes pain in the lower back due to stress in the ligaments on the spine, the discs, and the facet joints. The solution is to stretch the hamstrings, hip muscles, and spine by flattening the lumbar spine. Anyone affected by this common problem can find relief of low back pain by doing stretching exercises every day for fifteen minutes twice a day.

Excessive exercise is not necessary to stay healthy or live longer. When we take many risks or develop risky behaviors, we may damage our joints and discs or tear our ligaments. Recurrent injuries or pain indicates that the exercise you're engaging in is excessive. Repetitive sports injuries are common. The same is true if this happens at work. It is better to be safe than sorry. Violent and painful exercises are not necessary. Exercise should be enjoyable to be beneficial.

Another common problem with excessive exercise or repetitive movements is inflammation of the joints, tendons, ligaments, and small sacs in the joints known as bursa. Inflammation of these tissues can limit our activities, leading to pain and weakness of muscles. The first thing to do is to avoid excessive exercise. If this is not possible, a modified exercise is the solution. If pain continues, remember the acronym RICE (rest, ice, compression, and elevation) to get relief. This is a basic concept in sport-related injuries.

If this still is not sufficient, consultation with a doctor or specialist is recommended. The treatment may include rest, steroid injections, and NSAIDs like ibuprofen. I also recommend supplements to control inflammation. Turmeric powder, found in grocery stores in the spice section, is one. Sprinkle turmeric in your salads or cereal twice a day. Turmeric is also available in capsules that contain small amounts of pepper for better absorption. They are in vitamin shops under the name curcumin. Omega-3 every day can also reduce inflammation. People with knee or joint problems can add glucosamine since it appears to help to repair cartilage. Joint pain can be helped with another supplement called SAM-e, taken at 200 mg twice a day. Many supplements help to reduce pain without the need of narcotic analgesics.

As we age, we should exercise daily to maintain our strength and balance of all our physiological functions. We call this practice "conditioning." When we do not exercise, we develop a deconditioning syndrome. Folks in their eighties or beyond must exercise to avoid falls caused by weakness. Failure to do so may result in fractures and more weakness. Workouts help to condition muscles for more strenuous activities. Exercise not only helps the joints, ligaments, bones, and muscles to remain healthy, it also helps the brain to remain engaged and active. If a person does not use a muscle, he or she will lose use of it. (Use it or lose it!)

Remember to stretch before exercising. Stretching helps the muscles and ligaments get ready to exercise, increases flexibility, and improves posture. Physiologically, stretching helps to create a feeling of relaxation and diminishes stress.

How does exercise help to produce natural painkillers?

When we exercise, the body produces endorphins—which rhymes with morphin—to eliminate pain. Endorphins are natural painkillers that work like morphin to relieve pain. People who exercise for hours may experience some euphoria due to an "endorphin rush." This is the reason some athletes or football players do not feel pain when they are playing with an injury or fracture. The same is true when someone is involved in an accident. The release of endorphins minimizes the pain that is evident hours later when there are no more endorphins circulating. The body produces minute amounts of endorphins, but they are not sufficient to stop severe or chronic pain. Exercising regularly helps to relieve pain due to the production of natural endorphins. People who exercise have a higher threshold for pain than people who don't exercise. That is why people with back pain feel better when they exercise but worse when they are inactive or in bed.

Besides these natural painkillers, exercise increases the production of a protein known as BDNF, or brain-derived neurotrophic factor. This protein promotes neurogenesis, which is the production of new nerve cells in the brain to replace damaged areas or dying cells. This is what happens in individuals who have sustained strokes and brain injuries. My decades of experience helping to rehabilitate people with brain injuries have given me more insight about the plasticity of the brain and the improvement of cognitive function. I have seen patients who, ten years after a brain injury, have experienced significant improvement in their speech and cognitive functions with proper training and guidance and exercise.

How does exercise help to develop muscle mass?

As we age, we lose muscle mass; muscles become smaller, and we lose strength. This progressive weakness can be reversed with regular exercise. Studies indicate that a person with a sedentary lifestyle loses from 6 to 7 percent of muscle mass every decade. If a person exercises, the loss is limited to 2 to 3 percent per decade. By age sixty, a sedentary person has lost about 25 percent of muscle mass. An active person loses only 8 percent. Muscle mass loss is a consequence of inactivity. A person who is very active at age seventy-four may have similar muscle mass to a person who is forty and exercises periodically.

This is more proof of the "mind over matter" thought process. When you make up your mind and set a goal for yourself, your thoughts create a different set of values and behaviors that change your life. Developing an exercise regime to prevent muscle mass and deconditioning will help you to be as strong as a younger person. This is how you can modify unhealthy behaviors, look younger, and reverse aging.

How does exercise help maintain a normal weight?

You can keep your weight in check if you exercise regularly to burn excessive fat. Exercise is an effective way to lose the extra pounds you want to lose without any medications or appetite suppressants. When we eat too much food and particularly carbohydrates, we accumulate glycogen in the liver and muscles. Any excess of carbohydrates is accumulated as fat in fatty cells, in the abdomen and later in other parts of the body. When we exercise, we need to burn the glycogen in the liver and muscles before we begin to burn the fat in the fat deposits. Fasting helps to burn the glycogen and fats. Exercise accelerates the burning of both glycogen and fats.

My wife and I eat very light for two or three days after a dinner party. We like to enjoy the dinner or the wine and occasionally the dessert. We have a plan to deal with the calories and the weight gain. The plan is fasting and exercise. Sometimes, it may take a week to lose the excess weight before we return to our regular meal routine. If we exercise longer every day, we lose the excess weight in two to three days.

We check our weight on our scales without clothing before going to bed and in the morning to see the results. If the weight gain continues, the fasting diet and the exercise will continue until we return to our regular weight. Once we return to our normal weight, we eat a regular meal that includes salad with oil vinaigrette dressing, salmon or broiled fish, celery or broccoli, and water with lemon. We also increase the time we exercise every day to burn more calories and keep weight down and stable. I recommend this regimen as a way to lose weight and keep it from fluctuating every day. It also may help those who have lost considerable weight and want to develop a routine to prevent gaining weight again. I have found that this issue is very frustrating for many people who begin to regain lost weight. What is important is to have the discipline to incorporate healthy behaviors in your lifestyle like fasting and exercise.

Can exercise help to prevent the decline of functions as we age?

The short answer is yes. As we age, our physiological body functions decline year after year. This process begins by about age thirty and progresses gradually. Most of our functions roughly decline about 1 percent every year. This means that, after ten years, many organ functions have declined about 10 percent. Renal, lung, and muscular functions by age eighty are at about 50 percent of the function of age thirty. Bone loss increases with age. In women, the rate of loss is about 8 percent after age thirty every decade. This means that, by age eighty, a woman has experienced 40 percent bone loss. For men, the loss is lower, only 3 percent per decade after thirty. Heart function and cardiac output by age eighty also declines by 40 percent in a healthy person without coronary disease. In the presence of coronary disease, cardiac output by age eighty may decrease more depending on the damage to the heart. The brain also suffers decline. Exercise stimulates the production of serotonin and GABA, which lowers anxiety and increases memory capacity. A 2009 study from the University of Groningen in the Netherlands showed that building muscle mass leads to neurogenesis, the creation of new nerve cells, and angiogenesis, the creation of new vessels and increased blood flow. Blood flow declines by 50 percent by age eighty. It declines faster in people with atherosclerosis, diabetes, or peripheral vascular disease, leading to dementia and loss of many body functions. As we can see from these numbers, all organs have considerable function reserve when we are young. This reserve is gradually lost as we age. Regular exercise can reduce these losses. A study from the University of Utah found that just two minutes for every hour spent sitting dramatically reduces the risk of early death—by 33 percent. Another study from the University of Cambridge found that one hour of moderate exercise eliminates the risk of early death due to sedentary activity.

Klotho is a longevity protein found in the brain that helps to improve memory, cognitive function, language and visual and spatial intelligence. People who carry the gene that produces this protein usually score higher on IQ tests. Recent studies suggest that aerobic exercise helps to raise the levels of this protein. Some research also suggests that exercise may help decrease the effects of the ApoE4 gene and the formation of plaque responsible for a well-defined form of Alzheimer's disease.

Benefits of exercise

As a specialist in rehabilitation medicine, I learned early in my career that exercise helps to restore function and improve survival. As related in chapter 9's discussion on genetic and telomere research on longevity and DNA, during my early years of practice, I was involved in developing programs to improve heart function after heart attacks and coronary artery bypass surgery. Most of our patients were monitored with telemetry to assess the heart function during exercise. The results were remarkable. In many cases, a person had arrhythmias before exercising but had them disappear with exercise after a few weeks. Cardiac output improved to almost normal levels as well. These findings were confirmed by improvements in cardiac output and ejection fraction studies months later. My experience in cardiac rehabilitation was very helpful in designing exercise programs for people with strokes, orthopedic issues, and weight problems. I personally feel exercise is good in preventing the decline of our physiological functions, which diet alone cannot improve. Many studies have confirmed my observations. Dr. Kenneth Cooper at his Cooper Aerobics Center in Dallas conducted many studies demonstrating the benefits of aerobic exercise in cardiac function. Given the unavoidable natural decline of our body functions, cardiac output, and reserves, it is important to add exercise to our daily activities.

Exercise provides many benefits to our overall health. During exercise, our bodies produce myokines, which stimulate muscle growth, tissue repair and anti-inflammatory functions. Exercise improves blood flow in the heart, brain, muscle, and tissues. When we exercise, we bring more oxygen and nutrients to the tissues, helping to repair and remove damaged cells and toxic materials.

Exercise helps keep the mind alert. Patients who have had strokes and lost the neurons responsible for a given muscle function can regain the function through retraining. Keeping the brain active through exercise is a healthy function and behavior. We can influence the brain and intellect by repetitive activity. A pianist develops remarkable skills from stored movements in memory banks that are learned through repetitive motion. The same is true for dancers or skilled workers. Repetitive exercises help us to understand why it is beneficial to maintain skills that help to preserve and keep our memories healthy and prevent the development of Alzheimer's disease or memory problems as we age.

Exercise is one of the elements of my DRESS-SS prescription. It is possible to bring our diet and hormones to a perfect equilibrium. Without exercise, the body's physiological functions will continue to decline unless we introduce exercise as a means to decrease this natural loss of our reserves of all our physiological functions.

Exercise also has a positive influence on our sense of well-being, self-esteem, mood, sexual function, and happiness. As people age, many individuals become withdrawn, inactive, and depressed. Adding to this mix, the lack of exercise in these folks accelerate aging, with greater loss of physiological function. All this can be prevented by exercising regularly. The American College of Sports Medicine has developed guidelines detailing levels of exercise to maintain aerobic fitness and physical vigor in healthy aging adults. For more information about these exercise guidelines, you can visit their website at www.acsm.org.

Exercise has a positive effect on improving sleep and controlling stress, two other elements of my DRESS-SS prescription. Sexual activity also declines with age. Exercise has a positive benefit when it comes to sustaining levels of sexual function. Surveys have shown that running enhances the libido and lives of those who run regularly. In general, involvement in any sport activity and meaningful sexual relationships has positive benefits in all body functions and emotions.

My recommendation to anyone following my DRESS-SS prescription is to make exercise an essential and important part of your daily routine. Remember, you need regular exercise to prevent loss of muscle mass and strength after age thirty. Exercise should include strengthening and endurance (cardio) exercises. Ideally, you should exercise for one hour every day, but at a minimum one hour three times a week is beneficial to reverse the decline associated with aging. Exercise has positive effects on your brain, all your body functions to increase longevity, and your overall happiness. Exercise is better than medicines because it provides nutrients and oxygen to your cells. Exercise is there for you to enjoy; it is free, and you can get as much as you want to stay healthy, live longer, and reverse aging.

CHAPTER 5

S is for Stress and Stress Management

How can we define stress?

The definition of stress is "a psychophysical reaction to pressure on an individual from internal or external sources." Stress is both external and internal. External stress comes from our environment. Anything outside our bodies could be stressful. Our home, family, work, community, or government could be examples of external stressors. Internal stress comes from within. All our hopes, desires, expectations, relationships, dreams, negative feelings, fantasies, passions, and our responses to injuries or illness are examples of internal stressors. From the time we are born, stress surrounds us. Too much stress has a deleterious effect on our health and happiness.

Stress is part of life. However, too much stress is unhealthy. As a doctor, I feel most of people's illnesses and doctor visits are secondary to the stress in their daily lives. All living organisms are subject to some kind of stress. The stressor is the stimulus that causes stress. It can be positive or negative. The stressor can cause a form of acute or chronic stress. Acute stress occurs when we are suddenly affected by an unexpected situation that triggers a fight-or-flight response. Stressors come in all forms—a death in the family, an accident, a major financial failure, a bad diagnosis, or a serious illness. When a stressor continues for a long period, meaning weeks, months, or years, the stress becomes chronic and may lead to significant health problems.

Positive or good stress, also known as "eustress," is the type of stress that helps any individual to thrive or succeed. This type of stress helps people to become creative, inspire others, and enhance their lives and those of others. We can use this stress to our benefit. If properly guided with discipline and rest, it can be channeled into a creative force that allows us to win a game, pass an exam, graduate with honors, become an Olympic athlete, or become the champion of a cause.

To live longer, happier, and healthier, a person has to become aware of the stressors that are affecting his or her life. Knowing the enemy helps to deal with the problem. Modern life is stressful. We live very busy lives compared with our ancestors. We drive cars, fly planes, watch TV, and use iPhones. We are constantly bombarded by negative news. Tending to family, children, and loved ones, especially in the case of loss or separation, may be very demanding and add to our daily stress load. Our work could be very stressful. All these stressors are reasons we must pay more attention to the inner self to develop coping mechanisms and tools to deal with the stress of everyday life. One way to deal with this stress is resilience or an ability to adapt and persevere in the face of failure or adversity. Resilience is an important ingredient to cope with daily stress and failure, to succeed in life, and to achieve happiness. In *Living Longer and Reversing Aging*, I have emphasized the power of our thoughts to change and make choices. To be more resilient, you must change the way you think about failure and adversity.

How can we manage stress?

Developing coping mechanisms and resilience

Taking breaks, meditating, and sleeping well are good coping mechanisms to deal with our daily stress. In previous chapters, I emphasized the need to take breaks and sleep from seven to eight hours each night. These are ways to provide our bodies the time to recover from the stressors of the day and the production of cortisol and adrenaline, which may lead our bodies to exhaustion. Developing resilience is another way to cope with the stressors of daily life. You probably know someone who lost a member of the family or went bankrupt. The losses seem overwhelming. Some of them seem to accept the loss or failure and rise to move on and write another chapter in their lives. Their courage and determination is inspiring. In spite of the trauma, they look forward to finding new opportunities or solutions. They find meaning in failure and work hard to achieve new levels of success and loving relationships. It is our responsibility to take care of our bodies by giving them a chance to recover from the overwhelming stressors in our daily lives. With so many obligations, we sometimes forget about listening to the self. We should take time during the day to meditate and analyze whether overwhelming stress is worthy or necessary.

As a physician specialist in physical rehabilitation, I have seen many people who sustained overwhelming injuries resulting in quadriplegia or paralysis. Some may have sustained multiple fractures. All of them require extensive rehabilitation. It is rewarding to see how many of them rise to the challenge and work hard toward their recovery. I personally know and have treated patients who were paralyzed from the waist down and now are able to drive, have children, and have successful careers. They are examples of resilience and are very inspiring. You can learn the skills to help you overcome failure and stress in order to succeed in life. *Living Longer and Reversing Aging* offers you a prescription to change your lifestyle and grow in resilience. This is a prescription for a lifetime, not for a day or a week, and requires a lifetime commitment to change.

Chronic stress eventually will cause damage to your health. The excessive production of cortisol, adrenaline, and other brain hormones and neurotransmitters will cause damage to your nerve cells and organs. Hypertension, chronic anxiety, depression, insomnia, weight gain, diabetes, infections, and cancer are some of the consequences. These internal changes are good reasons to pay attention to your health and begin to make changes to improve your health and life span.

Scientists have demonstrated that stress affects the immune system as well. This is why we are more susceptible to colds, flu, and viral and bacterial infections when we're under too much stress. One of the reasons for this weak immune system is the elevated levels of cortisol present when we experience stress. Too much cortisol interferes with the immune response. Stress decreases our levels of cytokines, a substance that provides signals to the brain that the body is being attacked and becoming susceptible to damage by a virus or a bacteria. Acute stressors are unavoidable and should be promptly resolved. Allowing an acute stressor to become chronic is a mistake. Over time, chronic stress will become worse, and the toll on the body and the mind will be greater.

Practicing mindfulness meditation is a way to overcome negative feelings and anxiety. Buddhists practiced this type of meditation for thousands of years. This type of meditation brings peace and calmness to your mind. You need to become aware of your feelings and decide how to deal with them and with stress. You should ask yourself if negative feelings and the stress you are experiencing make you happy. If your answer is no, it is time to adjust your lifestyle. If you put aside your negative feelings while you meditate, you will get closer to the positive side of your feelings.

When you meditate, imagine that you have been transported to the heavens, where there is no hate, anger, jealousy, or stress. If you can transfer this feeling of joy during meditation to your daily life and stressful situations, you will experience greater happiness. This perhaps explains why we love dogs. They love and accept us even if we are angry, jealous, or hateful. Animals do not use their time or energy holding grudges. They are more concerned with survival than with being hateful or mad. Uncontrolled negative feelings and excess anxiety are human reactions and creations that have undermined our path toward greater happiness. When you meditate to enjoy a moment without negative feelings, you will realize the importance of happiness in your life.

What is mindfulness meditation?

I have recommended in this book the use of mindfulness meditation as a way to manage stress and anxiety. Many people may not have heard the phrase "mindfulness meditation" before and may wonder what it is all about. The concept of mindfulness is very simple. A person must focus on the moment at hand in a nonjudgmental way. When you use a mindfulness approach, your thoughts are directed to something you choose on purpose at that moment without judging whether the experience is good or bad.

Most people go from one thing to another without purpose. They act like sleepwalkers through life. They run from one action to another. Women appear to have multiple antennas and have many projects or worries at the same time. Levels of anxiety and depression are higher in women who have many things in their mind. With child rearing, health problems, work, spousal issues, financial concerns, and family problems, many women have no time to think about themselves or take a break or time to think about their own feelings and lifestyles. They wake up in the morning and start the day on automatic pilot, repeating the same routines they did the day before and the day before that. They often do not even remember what they did the day before and don't realize their bad diets and behaviors are harmful and unhealthy to them and the entire family.

Any minor discomfort, rejection, or negative event may trigger a negative train of thoughts, making their anxiety worse. These concerns and negative thoughts in many people, and particularly in women, cause the brain function to speed up without control, rendering it unable to unwind at night, relax, and slow down the thoughts before going to bed. Naturally, they have difficulty falling asleep. If insomnia sets in, they are tired and without energy the next morning. Day after day, the increased stress and sleep deprivation makes life more difficult.

Often this strains relationships with loved ones, including the spouse and children. Job performance and productivity may be affected to the point of being reprimanded by superiors. In an era of hyperconnectivity, most people remain constantly connected to their iPhones or iPads. Messaging and emailing is now an addiction. People have no time to speak or pay attention without looking at their devices to check for messages, Twitter, or email. This is causing people to become disconnected with their feelings, coworkers, and environment. Many corporate workers find no time to take breaks to rest their minds. People are having difficulties disconnecting from their phones. In fact, many tech companies are using mindfulness meditation to help workers to focus on the present to give their brains a break. Doing this helps to free up mental space, improves creativity, and inspires deep thinking. You can find apps about mindfulness meditation on iTunes. One app called Headspace offers free content and sells videos that explain how to meditate.

Mindful meditation has a long tradition in Buddhism. A scientist known as Jon Kabat-Zinn, a PhD in molecular biology in the 1970s, promoted this form of meditation. Since then, many universities and medical centers have accepted and adopted his technique. There are multiple apps on the internet to guide you to learn mindfulness meditation, as well as muscle relaxation training to reduce anxiety and stress. Corporations use mindfulness meditation to help workers to relax and concentrate on the present. There are now many instructors who teach and courses called mindfulness-based stress reduction (MBSR). I have personally used mindfulness meditation in my pain management practice since the early 1980s.

During the sessions, patients with chronic pain learn to manage their pain by using meditation and behavioral therapy techniques. It helps them relax and concentrate on one task. In the beginning, I used biofeedback training and muscle relaxation techniques using EMG biofeedback training. When the muscles were completely relaxed, people with chronic pain were able to go into deep relaxation and find relief of their pain for hours without the need of analgesics. Practicing these techniques helped them to go without any opioids for days.

Over the years, I found that, to be effective, mindfulness meditation should be practiced for ten to thirty minutes a day. It can offer a level of deep muscle relaxation and an unwinding of the brain activity. In a state of relaxation, an individual stops the release of cortisol and adrenaline, which increase the levels of stress. I personally feel that those individuals in highly stressful jobs like the military are in great danger of developing harm to their bodies and minds by the constant release of cortisol and adrenaline. Learning mindfulness meditation should help the military in combat to reduce the level of stress and concentrate on the task. No wonder so many veterans suffer from PTSD (post-traumatic stress disorder). The same can be said of businesses where stress is very toxic. I recommend that anyone who is under stress should practice mindfulness meditation and muscle relaxation. If you need more help, find the apps for guidance.

Practicing mindfulness helps you to recognize you are on autopilot and allows you to look at yourself in a more positive way in order to control your feelings and organize your life based on priorities. To do this, take time and sit down or lie down with your eyes closed and focus on the moment. Think about your body and feelings. Become aware of what makes you unhappy or why you are feeling sad, tired, or stressed or are in a bad mood. Leave aside for a while all the other thoughts that keep you on autopilot. Begin to plan and make good choices to feel better physically and emotionally. When you use your mind to meditate and find solutions to your problems, you are practicing mindfulness and raising your resilience.

One way to start practicing mindfulness meditation is to direct your thoughts to a current experience. If you are sitting, notice your environment around you—the sounds, the people, and the music. Then think about your body and how you feel. Think about your posture, your joints, and the contact with the chair or the floor. Take a deep breath and exhale. You will begin to feel relaxed and in control of your body and breathing. This is a moment for you to enjoy and connect with yourself. If you have a fruit or a candy, look at it and feel it with your fingers and tongue. Then taste it. Without swallowing, feel the taste and pleasure before, while, and after you swallow. Repeat this with another piece, swallowing slowly to enjoy the feeling and exploring all your senses—sight, touch, smell, taste, and sound.

As you learn to focus, you will focus on your feelings. You should feel that you are in charge and in control of your feelings. Don't look at yourself as a victim, since this will increase your level of stress and affect your capacity to change and become more resilient. In the next meditation session, you will focus on what makes you happy and what you can do to achieve greater happiness. If you bring positive thoughts, you can plan how to achieve your goal. Take small steps before you go a greater distance. If you feel that you need to write what you are going to do, do it now. Set up priorities and deadlines. As you get used to focusing on your thoughts, you will begin to see changes. Your life is no longer on autopilot because you are now taking time to use your mind to direct your actions and manage your feelings in a positive direction. You are in control of your thoughts and feelings. You can change your thinking style to improve your life and enjoy better health and longer longevity.

If you experience great emotional distress and are unable to focus your feelings to find solutions, you may need professional help or counseling. A trained professional can help you to improve your resilience and coping mechanisms. Don't hesitate or procrastinate if you need someone to help you to get out of this dark maze. Humility is an asset. Failure is a human experience and an opportunity to learn and become a better person. In sports, the best teams lost many games before they became better. The same is true with people. We all have different kinds of painful experiences that help us to grow and become more human and enjoy life. As a doctor, I see human failure and illness all the time. I feel better when I can help someone to overcome their trauma or loss of function from serious illnesses or injury. You may need family support, but you are the one who should make the decisions to change your thinking in order to relieve overwhelming stress. If you meditate, you may come to this conclusion through mindfulness meditation. This skill is a way to develop a coping mechanism to deal with stress, increase resilience, and deal with chronic pain and family problems.

Mindfulness meditation is also a way to practice muscle relaxation training to overcome stress, eliminate phobias, and rid yourself of unexplained fears. In my practice, I recommend this to people with a fear of flying in an airplane. I recommend that they relax on a couch, close their eyes, and see themselves at the airport ready to board the plane. As they feel comfortable in their seats, they should see themselves relaxed and free of fear. As the plane begins to climb, they should feel relaxed and free of negative thoughts. This should continue until they see the plane landing. Practicing this form of behavioral therapy and mindfulness meditation several times a day for ten to thirty minutes helps to overcome anxiety and fears, preparing your brain to think differently. The same can be done with any type of fear or stress. This practice is healthier than becoming dependent on medications like benzodiazepines.

Chapter 3, "R is for Rest," is dedicated to the rest part of my DRESS-SS prescription. I recommend that you review this chapter if you have too much stress. Taking a break or a moment in our busy lives to know where we are and where we are going is an important part of finding purpose and directing our actions in life. We are physical, emotional, intellectual, and spiritual beings, but we take no time to think about it. We become physical, emotional, or intellectual doers and impose on ourselves tasks and activities without any breaks to become aware of what we are doing or where we are going. Mindfulness meditation changes lives for the better since it raises your resilience. It provides time and space to think about our journey and purpose in life.

Mindfulness meditation is like a rest stop or a pause button in a long trip. We all need to stop to stretch, relax, exercise, eat, and take care of our physiological functions to continue the journey. You should press your pause button every day, even if it is just for a few minutes. This break will be beneficial to your health, if you want to improve your health, grow happier, and live longer.

How do internal stressors affect us positively or negatively?

We mentioned above that internal stressors could be positive or negative. Positive thinking helps to relieve stress. If you want a life full of joy and happiness, you must change your attitude in a positive way, or nothing good will happen. A positive psychological well-being must be your goal in life. Negative thinking triggers negative feelings of anger, hate, jealousy, and distrust. When those negative feelings are projected onto others, there is always a negative reaction. Arguments may ensue, leading to confrontation and increased anger. Physiologically, there is increased release of adrenaline and cortisol. If this is your situation in a marriage, you can understand the high level of stress you have every day. Many of these conflicts may start by a false belief or impression. Your spouse may be thinking you are having an affair because you are not talking enough, look worried, and have a different attitude. Sometimes this happens without any foundation. The stressor is a negative thought from feelings of insecurity that arise from bad experiences as a child or previous failed relationships. It is imperative that you become aware of the quality of your thoughts. The reality is that anything a human being creates starts with a thought that is followed by an action. Actions generate reactions by others around us. Misunderstandings by negative thoughts could be devastating to you and the family. Delusional thinking can be interpreted as reality and may lead to bad choices.

As a doctor, I want you to realize that the life you want for yourself depends on the thoughts you make all the time and how these thoughts can be transformed into something positive, meaningful, and real. When you focus your thoughts on something you want, you are calling these thoughts into existence. When you think about a better paying job or a less stressful job, your mind is creating a new reality for yourself. If you pursue what these thoughts are telling you, you will act and will make a choice and find what you want. If you feel better after getting what you want, you may wonder, Why did it take me so long to make a change and improve my life for the better? Thinking positively helps you to deal with stress. Use this approach to reduce stress and improve the quality of your life. Nothing will happen unless you guide your thoughts toward positive feelings and happiness.

When you think you want a vacation on a beautiful island, it becomes reality the moment you buy the tickets and arrive at this distant place. The same is true when you want a house or a car. You always dream about something you want, but it will not happen until you turn these thoughts into reality. You attract what you want.

If you hang out with bad friends who use drugs and alcohol, you are attracting bad company, and eventually you will end up like them. Over time, when your life becomes a wreck, you will wonder how and when you made this mistake. The answer is simple. It was the dreadful day your thoughts attracted such bad company. This was the day the quality of your life began to decline, and your stress levels went sky-high. If there is too much stress in your life now, you can change this situation if you meditate and focus on your thoughts right now. You have the power to create a new life for yourself with positive thoughts. You don't need medicines or visits to a psychiatrist. What you need is action and a positive attitude to reduce the stress on your life and be happy every day of your life.

You may have experienced feelings from people you meet every day. You may have experienced sadness, anger, jealousy, or hate and reacted with similar energy towards someone. You must become aware how this positive or negative energy is affecting you. Negative or positive thoughts affect your life in many ways. Negativity is associated with anxiety and depression. The balance of thoughts should always be in favor of positive thoughts. When you become aware of how you react, you will begin to understand why you react that way and of who and what is causing you stress. At this point, you will become aware of how powerful or weak you are and how you can confront and change your life and everything around you.

When our minds and hearts are full of positive thoughts and feelings, most likely we are ready to project a positive attitude and face any potential conflict. Positive thoughts and attitudes can shape your lifestyle for the better, and you will enjoy better health and less stress. This happens when you channel your thoughts to be positive and happy. Positive thinking raises the levels of serotonin, a hormone that helps you feel joy and happiness. Negative thinking decreases the levels of serotonin, leading to depression. The treatment for depression is directed to raising the serotonin levels. Most antidepressants act to raise serotonin in the brain. To prevent depression, a person must develop a positive attitude and positive thoughts, or he or she will relapse into depression again.

Love is a powerful feeling that also helps humans reduce stress and achieve happiness and is the basis for anything you want to achieve. If you want to feel better every day, you need to attract and project love. By doing so, you will create positive thoughts and feelings for others, which will help you to fulfill your goal of moving toward happiness. If you are depressed, it is very likely you have many negative thoughts and your serotonin levels are depleted. When this situation becomes chronic, you may need an antidepressant to elevate your serotonin levels to balance the neurotransmission in your brain.

As a rule, nothing good comes from a negative mind. If this is your situation, most likely your family or peers will see you as a troubled person, projecting an image or attitude full of anger, indifference, hate, or isolation. You may have difficulty getting along with others, complaining frequently about anyone and everything and displaying a sour or negative mood. Most people want to distance themselves from such a negative and depressed person. Negativism leads to anger and bad relations with family and coworkers. To excuse this attitude, a negative person begins to blame others, such as parents, family, spouse, children, coworkers, politicians, or the government, for his or her problems. An attitude of self-pity develops to justify the negative behavior. Negative feelings associated with anger may become dangerous and threatening. Anyone going through this stage must find professional help.

Making positive choices can end destructive behaviors and negative attitudes. If you are unhappy with your job, you should find another job. If the problem is more emotionally draining, such as dealing with a child with special needs or a loved one who is ill, you must learn how to manage the stress through meditation, taking care of your body, seeking spirituality, and garnering emotional support and love from others in similar situations. You might even consider joining a support group. At all times, you should choose love over hate or bitterness. Love is a powerful feeling that will lead you to happiness and less stress in your life. You have the freedom to choose, but choices have consequences. Good choices will be rewarded, and bad choices will be punished.

There are situations when a loved one is chronically ill with a disease like cancer, and there seems to be no way to find relief from the stressful situation. You may think there is nothing much you can do, but you are wrong. You have your creative mind and thoughts. They will guide you to the best outcome if you put your mind into it. Spirituality, a sense of purpose, optimism, compassion, gratitude, and love provide a path to find some relief. If you are the only caregiver, you should take care of yourself. Otherwise, your health will be affected, and your loved ones will be without anyone to take care of their needs.

Talking to friends and family or support groups may help to relieve stress. Try mindfulness meditation every day. Today you can find meditation apps that will help you to relieve stress and guide you to feel better. You can talk to a pastor, a preacher, or a counselor for guidance. There are many examples of people who were lost and found a purpose in life and made good choices that eventually helped them to overcome their sorrow, negative thoughts, anxiety, and depression.

There are many stories of people who went through difficult times but had faith in God or a higher power. Praying as part of a spiritual life helps as well. As a doctor, I have found that, spirituality played an important role in helping people with serious medical problems and depression to cope with stress and find peace and healing.

Humor is also a positive way to cope with stress. It helps us to relax and forget our negative feelings or problems for a while. When humor is positive, you feel better. Positive thoughts and laughter help to recharge your emotional batteries and help you leave the deep hole of anxiety and depression. Meditate, exercise, take a walk, sing a song, call a friend, help someone in need, or volunteer your time to help others in need in your community. Once you can get a handle on making good and positive choices, your level of stress will subside.

The person who moves without purpose from one action to another as if on autopilot must stop, take a break to think about living in the present, and meditate on what is to be done. Use your mind to change your life and future.

Do not sacrifice greater happiness for a little happiness. Workaholics are never truly happy. They feel more work is necessary to achieve something, and when the work is done, they still feel no satisfaction. Money, fame, and success do not necessarily result in happiness. Many people who devote themselves to work sacrifice relationships with family, spouse, and children; eventually they will find themselves unhappy and unfulfilled. Enjoy the moment, live in the present, and practice mindfulness meditation.

This book is a guide to finding a path to reach happiness. Review each chapter and you will find the way to become healthier physically and emotionally. Become aware of your environment and emotions to make positive choices. Focus your thoughts on the present and the real world in front of you. When you do this, you become more productive, and your actions become more joyful and rewarding. Love and happiness should become the nutrients for the soul. You deserve it. Use my prescription to keep living a healthier lifestyle, and you will find more and greater happiness every day.

Other causes of physical stress

How can hormone imbalances lead to stress?

Stress is essentially a disruption of the normal balance or equilibrium in the physiology of our bodies. This equilibrium is known as homeostasis. Many hormones are produced in the hippocampus and have an effect on the target organs, like the ovaries, adrenal glands, thyroid, and testicles. They stimulate the production of hormones in these organs. In turn, the hormones from these organs decrease the production of hormones from the hippocampus to maintain equilibrium. When this homeostasis is disrupted, different kinds of symptoms develop. Checking the levels of hormones and replacing deficiencies can bring the system back to equilibrium.

Most people are unaware of these deficiencies that are responsible for early aging and health problems. These hormonal disruptions are sources of internal stress. This internal stress, compounded with external stress in an individual, magnifies any already existing symptoms that may lead to anxiety, depression, or panic attacks. That is why it is important to pay attention to the internal causes of stress when our external stressors are under control. In my experience, people who keep the homeostasis of their hormonal system in equilibrium look younger and healthier. They are also happier. Estrogen and testosterone help to reverse aging.

Estrogen, a female hormone that begins to decline during menopause, causes hot flashes, skin changes, loss of hair, and premature aging. The skin loses its moisture. Over time, wrinkles ensue and become prominent. Bone loss or osteopenia develops gradually, which leads to osteoporosis if left unattended. This is why many women are very susceptible to fractures beginning in their sixties. If there is no family history of ovarian or breast cancer, estrogens are recommended, since they help keep the body healthy, improve libido, prevent premature aging, slow osteoporosis, and prevent fractures.

Estrogen also helps to decrease internal stress associated with the deficiency of this hormone and the symptoms related to this gradual change. Women may also experience deficiencies of testosterone, resulting in decreased sexual drive. It is common for women to experience a loss of sexual drive and intimacy as they age. This loss in sexual drive causes friction in a marriage when women lose their desire for an intimate sexual relationship. This could lead to stress, but it can be relieved simply by asking a doctor to check for estrogen and testosterone levels.

Not all women respond well to estrogens during menopause. Some may experience severe hot flashes and changes in behavior. The stress from these symptoms raises the levels of cortisol and adrenaline responsible for the symptoms and persistent stress. Medication to relieve anxiety or antidepressants may help to provide relief. Supplements like GABA, Gotu kola and Bacopa may help to minimize the symptoms. Estrogens and testosterone are covered in more detail in chapter 7.

In men, low testosterone, or low T, is one of the causes of ED (erectile dysfunction). As the testosterone levels begin to decrease, usually by age fifty, many men begin to experience ED secondary to low testosterone levels. If a deficiency is present, an appropriate dosage of testosterone can improve sexual drive and eliminate the stress in the relationship.

If, in addition to hormonal balance, you practice mindfulness meditation, manage stress through positive thinking, make a commitment to eating a healthy diet, get enough rest and sleep, and create an environment of love and happiness the telomeres in your chromosomes will remain healthy. Some studies suggest that our telomeres, the small cuffs at the ends of chromosomes, can actually grow longer with these practices, increasing our life spans. It is your choice to live better and longer and look younger and healthier. As described before, it is the mind, through your positive thoughts, good choices, and attitude that has the most important effect on the quality of life you want for yourself.

What other factors contribute to our stress?

Besides hormone homeostasis imbalances, our bodies are constantly bombarded by free radicals, which damage the cells and our DNA and cause inflammation. These free radicals are also internal stressors that contribute to our overall stress, premature aging, and damage of our DNA, often resulting in cancer. When we experience stress, our bodies also produce cortisol and epinephrine. Cortisol and epinephrine are produced in the adrenal glands upon the direction of a hormone produced in the hippocampus in the brain. These two hormones will signal the immune system to release cytokines to promote inflammation, preparing the white cells to be ready for an impending attack. The problem is that, when there are external factors triggering stress, the body is subjected to a constant bombardment of cytokines, which causes an inflammatory response. Any time we have inflammation of a tissue, other chemicals that elicit pain are released as well. Often people with high levels of stress complain of pain. Headaches, muscle aches, joint or bone pain, or stomachache are common when somebody is under chronic stress. Stress is the root of many painful conditions, such as fibromyalgia or unexplained pain in the absence of tissue injury or damage.

Eliminating the internal and external stressors provides relief of chronic pain. This is why using meditation, biofeedback, muscle relaxation training, and behavioral therapy can help people feel better. A balanced diet, antioxidants, omega-3, rest, relaxation, and supplements are also very helpful. Antioxidants in fruits like blueberries help to neutralize the free radicals that may damage the DNA of the cells that in turn may become cancerous. Recent studies have demonstrated how the metabolism of sugars at the mitochondrial level produces high levels of free radicals, which damage the DNA. These studies suggest that excessive levels of sugars in diets and the high levels of free radicals may be the cause for many cancers. It is fair to say that a diet rich in carbohydrates creates an internal stressor at the cellular level, with possible serious consequences and damage to the DNA.

What is the best way to control anxiety?

In general, I do not recommend antianxiety medications or antidepressants. They create dependency and affect memory. Xanax, also known by its generic name, alprazolam, is very addictive, like most benzodiazepines. Recent studies show that it affects memory in people over sixty and is one of the leading causes of Alzheimer's. Antidepressants may help to control severe anxiety, depression, and sleep problems, but they have side effects. A psychiatrist or neurologist should prescribe them only for short periods. I have found over many years of practice that mindfulness meditation and many supplements help anxiety and avoid dependency on drugs. Many of these supplements are botanicals from herbs used for hundreds of years in India, China, and other countries. They are effective and have minimal side effects.

Big pharmaceutical companies, through government regulations, do not allow any manufacturer to tell you these supplements are effective. They face penalties for marketing their products for specific conditions. Based on my experience as a doctor and patient feedback, many supplements work very well. This is so important in preventing people from becoming dependent on medications that are extremely addictive and are causing significant public health problems. GABA is a natural neurotransmitter in the brain that helps to relieve anxiety and provides a soothing and calming effect. It comes in fast-acting tablets available in supplement stores. Gotu kola is a botanical that is very effective in managing stress and anxiety. A product from Nature's Way and other manufacturers is available in capsules of 475 mg and should be taken twice each day.

Adrenal health is important to relieve stress. The adrenal glands are located on the top of the kidneys and secrete cortisol, adrenaline, estrogen and testosterone, and DHEA. When there is a perceived threat, the adrenal glands produce adrenaline first to increase the heart rate and allow more blood to go to the muscles and brain to run or fight. This way, the muscles and brain get more oxygen, which is the "gas" to keep the brain and muscles ready to act. Adrenaline raises the blood pressure. In the short run, this rush of adrenaline is not hurtful. The problem begins when this release becomes chronic. When this happens, the blood pressure rises most of the time and heart rate increases, causing palpitations or dangerous arrhythmias. When this becomes prolonged for days and months or most of the time, a person is in a state of chronic stress, which is reinforced by elevated levels of cortisol as well. Cortisol is a steroid hormone produced in the adrenal gland to help the liver to convert stored energy into sugar, which is rapidly released in to the bloodstream. The production of cortisol and adrenaline depletes the adrenal cortex of these hormones.

A product from Gaia Herbs containing holy basil and Siberian *Rhodiola* extracts is very useful to manage anxiety associated with high levels of cortisol. My patients report good relief of anxiety with this product. Some other products I found effective are Ashwagandha and Bacopa. Bacopa deserves special attention since it also helps memory and cognition. This herb has been used in India for more than three thousand years and is one the herbs in Indian Ayurvedic medicine described in Vedic texts for their properties to enhance comprehension, learning, and memory. Children in India use Bacopa to enhance learning. It comes in teas, syrups, capsules, and tinctures. Elderly people should consider its use if they are beginning to experience memory problems or possibly Alzheimer's disease. Another herb that is effective for anxiety is *Echinacea angustifolia* root extract, which is available in tablets and teas.

CHAPTER 6

S is for Sleep

We spend a third of our lives sleeping. Sleeping the right amount of time keeps us alive, healthy, and young. People who suffer from insomnia and sleep deprivation age faster and die prematurely, according to Judith Carroll, PhD, in a study presented June 10 in Seattle, Washington, at SLEEP 2015, the 29th annual meeting of the Associated Professional Sleep Societies. Their immune systems decline faster, resulting in more illnesses and poor health. When we sleep at night, we give our bodies an opportunity to become restful and refreshed, stronger, and healthier. Sleeping well is how our bodies repair damage done during the day by injury, a stressful environment, or psychological stress.

During sleep, all our tissues and cells are in a constant state of repair. Our bodies produce several hormones during sleep that repair and rejuvenate our bodies. Growth hormone is one important hormone released that gives our bodies more energy to repair cellular damage. This hormone stimulates the cells to promote the use of amino acids throughout the cell membranes and increases the rate of protein synthesis to repair tissues and promote wound healing.

While we sleep, levels of cortisol and adrenaline drop to relieve stress. We know the length of our telomeres decreases with age, so deep and refreshing sleep is necessary to protect the telomeres in our chromosomes and keep us living longer and feeling younger. Since sleep is our "time out" for cellular repair and release of growth hormone, we should make deep and refreshing sleep an important part of a healthy lifestyle. In fact, we cannot survive more than a week without sleep, while we can survive weeks without food.

To live longer and look younger and healthier, an adult needs from seven to eight hours of sleep. I recommend eight hours to everybody, particularly if you are very active or have a very stressful day. Skimping on sleep is foolish and eventually will catch up with you. The brain keeps an accounting of the hours we sleep. People who lack proper amounts of sleep feel tired and weak during the day. Children need more hours of sleep than adults do. Teenagers may need ten hours to feel fresh and capable of carrying out an active life of sports and intellectual and emotional development. Infants require fourteen hours of sleep. The levels of growth hormone in children are higher to maintain a developing and growing body. It is a mistake for parents to allow children to skip sleep for slumber parties or similar activities. The damage done to their bodies by interrupting the normal circadian cycles and hormone processes could cause serious problems to a child who is in a constant state of development. People working graveyard shifts disrupt the circadian cycle and the release of growth hormone, which can eventually result in many health problems.

The Sleeping Cycle

During the day, our brains are in a constant state of activity. An electroencephalogram shows many beta waves at a high frequency when we are awake. Like our hearts, the greater our intellectual activity or stress, the higher the rate of waves. At night, or when we rest, the rate begins to decrease. When we go to sleep, our brain waves decelerate through five stages. Phases I to IV are known as non-REM (rapid eye movement). Phase V is characterized by rapid eye movements. This is the dream phase, or REM sleep.

Phase I begins when we feel sleepy and want to go to bed. This stage may last five to ten minutes. During phase II, we fall asleep. This stage may last from forty to fifty minutes. The rate of alpha waves decreases, and the body is more relaxed. As we descend into a deeper sleep, we enter into delta sleep, or very deep sleep. The brain at stage three is very calm and the body relaxed. The waves at this stage are called delta waves and are very slow. This is the most important stage of the sleep cycle. It is during this sleep phase that the body makes the most important repairs, releasing hormones, including growth hormone. Cortisol and epinephrine levels drop significantly at this point to reduce any stress. If we achieve delta sleep, we will feel refreshed the following day. This stage lasts between twenty and thirty minutes. If we wake up before reaching this stage, we are going to feel tired the following day. Reaching delta sleep is the most important goal for attaining better health, looking younger, and living longer. After phase III, the rate of the brain waves begins to increase gradually for about twenty to thirty minutes. We are still in deep refreshing sleep at phase IV of the sleep cycle.

When we reach phase V, we enter REM sleep. This is the stage where we begin to dream. Allegorically, it is like going to the movies to see the greatest and most mysterious show on earth. From the moment we go to bed, we have been descending a stairway and going deeper and deeper into a state of sleep before entering REM sleep. Once in this stage, brain waves increase in frequency, and memory banks become more active; breathing becomes heavier; and we use more oxygen. This phase lasts about twenty minutes. Many authors write books and stories about what we see and dream during this fascinating stage of the cycle. That is why REM sleep is so mysterious and intriguing. The entire cycle, from I to V, may be as short as 80 minutes or as long as 120 minutes. This cycle will repeat four or five times a night.

A normal and healthy person should go through all these stages every night without problems in order to stay healthy, keep a strong immune system, look younger, and live longer. If any of these stages is too short or impaired, the body and the mind will eventually pay the price. People working graveyard shifts are in a constant deficit since they do not go through the cycles at night when their circadian rhythms demand it. Many people who work at night or sleep fewer than seven hours feel tired and even exhausted. Even if a person sleeps during the day, the circadian cycle is impaired. Attempting to change a cycle that developed over millions of years of evolution is futile.

Insomnia is one the greatest problems for millions of people and the source of accidents, stress, weak immune systems, and chronic pain. People suffering from fibromyalgia usually have severe insomnia. The same is true of people with chronic headaches. To develop good sleeping habits, we should go to bed no later than 10:00 p.m.

About 10:00 p.m., the brain begins to slow down, and we begin to enter phase II of the sleeping cycle. About this time, our levels of melatonin begin to reach a level that makes us sleepy and tells us it is time to go to bed. Melatonin is a hormone produced in the pituitary gland in the brain. It is a powerful antioxidant and very important to achieve good and refreshing sleep. If we travel across different time zones, our circadian rhythm is off. The same may happen if we go to bed late after a party or a business meeting. If you have an important meeting the following day, you must sleep a minimum of seven hours that night. If your rhythm is off, I recommend taking from 3 to 5 mg of melatonin at least two hours before going to sleep. It takes time for melatonin to be absorbed and reach sufficient levels to induce sleep. If you do not have enough melatonin in your system, you will not reach delta sleep, the most relaxing and refreshing sleep. Without delta or deep sleep, our bodies begin to fail, and our immune systems weaken. Inflammation becomes chronic, pain becomes worse, aging accelerates, and our life span shortens. Deep sleep must be a daily goal and is essential for a healthy lifestyle.

What activities or factors affect our sleep patterns?

Our modern lives are inundated with the use of phones, computers, and television. It becomes very important to prepare for sleep every night. In the evening, we need to dim the lights to stimulate the production of melatonin, decrease many stimulating activities, and avoid bright computer and TV screens since the light reduces the production of melatonin. I do not recommend alcohol before going to bed. Initially, it may make you sleepy, but you may wake up hours later unable to sleep because of the low levels of melatonin in your brain. If you have trouble falling asleep, try to relax and dim the lights. Take valerian tea and 3 to 5 mg of melatonin. I do not recommend sleeping pills since they may interfere with your sleep the following nights, and they are habit forming. Occasionally, if you have a very important meeting the following day and have a hard time falling asleep, you may take 5 mg of Ambien to reach deep sleep. I do not recommend Valium or any benzodiazepines since they are habit forming.

If you have trouble breathing at night, your doctor may request a sleep test overnight, to evaluate whether you have sleep apnea. Sleep apnea causes hypoxia or oxygen deprivation of the brain due to a nasal or upper airway obstruction. People with sleep apnea snore and develop cognitive problems, hypertension, heart disease, and obesity. Obstructive sleep apnea also may be a factor in the development of Alzheimer's disease and dementia.

My wife and I usually sleep from seven to eight hours every night. I consider this practice one of the main reasons we are very healthy. I feel that a good night of sleep provides us with a good dose of growth hormone to repair cells and keep our immune systems strong. I also feel that a good night of sleep keeps us younger and may be part of the reason we look younger than our chronological ages. It is my opinion that a good night's sleep is rejuvenating and one of the main keys to living longer and healthier.

Researchers in the United Kingdom have found that cognitive behavioral therapy helps to improve insomnia. The *JAMA Psychiatry* journal also reported that people with insomnia might benefit from cognitive behavior therapy. I agree with those reports. The less medication used to improve sleep deprivation, the better. I prefer a well-balanced diet, herbs, supplements, exercise, and balanced nutrition and hormones to correct this chronic disorder. People with sleep disorders suffer from a chronic deficiency of growth hormone secreted by the pituitary during delta (deep) sleep. The limited amount of this hormone in those with sleep disorders leads to chronic tiredness, persistent headaches, and muscle and joint pain. People with chronic insomnia suffer from fibromyalgia. In my opinion, this is a syndrome resulting from a chronic growth hormone deficiency. Cognitive behavior therapy makes a lot of sense because it slows down the brain waves through cognitive training and exercises. While at rest, a person may begin to learn how to decelerate the brain activity before falling asleep.

What is insomnia?

Insomnia is defined as a complaint of disturbed sleep in the presence of an adequate opportunity and circumstance for sleep. The complaint may consist of difficulty initiating sleep, difficulty maintaining sleep, waking up too early, and/or nonrestorative or poor quality sleep. For the diagnosis of an insomnia disorder to be made, the difficulty with sleep must have a negative impact on daily function.

Insomnia is classified as either primary or comorbid. Primary insomnia implies that no other cause of sleep disturbance has been identified. Comorbid insomnia is more common and is most often associated with psychiatric disorders (for example, depression, anxiety, or substance use disorders); medical disorders (for example, cardiopulmonary disorders, neurologic disorders, or chronic somatic complaints that result in sleep disruption); medications; and other primary sleep disorders (for example, obstructive sleep apnea or restless legs syndrome). Comorbid insomnia does not suggest that other condition(s) "cause" insomnia, but rather that insomnia and the other condition(s) co-occur and may each warrant clinical attention and treatment.

Insomnia is a worldwide problem. It is estimated that sleep disorders affect from 50 to 70 million Americans, according to the National Institute of Health. The effects of this disorder become worse as people grow older. Opening the airway, either by nasal or sinus surgery, saline solution sprays, or vasoconstrictor nasal sprays, helps those with nasal congestion caused by mechanical problems in the nose and sinus cavities. New and smaller CPAP devices provide more oxygen to people with OSA (obstructive sleep apnea) and provide for better portability and comfort. OSA carries serious health consequences when left untreated. Any person with OSA should be advised to lose weight, if obesity is a risk factor. A person should consider a lap-band procedure or a gastric bypass if he or she is unable to lose weight.

To evaluate why you are experiencing insomnia, I recommend that you assess carefully your daily habits, your behaviors, and your use of medications and foods that may be affecting your sleep patterns.

Some behaviors and habits that may impair sleep include:

- Napping frequently during the day or before going to sleep
- Taking sleeping aids, Ambien, or benzodiazepines at night
- Taking diet pills, stimulants, or amphetamines
- Spending too much time in bed during the day
- Getting insufficient daytime exercise and mental activity to keep the body and mind stimulated
- Exercising late in the evening in forms that raise levels of serotonin and endorphins to stimulate your brain
- Getting insufficient bright light exposure during the day and too much light in the evening
- Taking excess caffeine or other stimulants, particularly in the evening
- Consuming alcohol in the evening
- Smoking in the evening
- Eating late heavy dinners and too many sugary snacks in the evening or before going to sleep
- Watching television or using the computer or working with too much light in the evening
- Having too much daily stress during the day and anxiety in the evening in anticipation of sleep

- Clock watching
- Failing to deal with environmental factors, such as the room being too warm, too noisy, or too bright or bad mattresses or pillows and uncomfortable beds
- Sleeping with pets on the bed or in the bedroom
- Sleeping next to partners who snore and are noisy
- Taking medications that may affect sleep

These are some suggestions to begin to eliminate factors affecting a good deep, refreshing sleep. Remember that the body begins to produce, in the evening, melatonin, a hormone that tells the brain it's time to go to sleep. Blue lights from fluorescent lights and LED lights in the evening decrease the production of melatonin and may cause macular degeneration, resulting in vision loss. If you work on your computer until too late at night, you will not have enough melatonin to reach a deep refreshing sleep. Don't use your computer, iPad, or iPhone too long at night.

I recommend using a blocker or dimming the screen light to decrease the light reaching your eyes. Apple launched Night Shift in iOS version 9, and Android Verizon 6, has a blue light filter. For desktop monitors, there is a program called f.flux that helps to block blue light. A better program is Iris, which can be obtained at http://iristech.co/iris-mini/. Dim the lights of your home every evening to allow your pituitary to make more melatonin. Another way to block blue light is to use blue light blocking glasses after the sunset. If you have problems falling asleep, I recommend using from 3 to 5 mg of melatonin two hours before you go to bed every night, to restore your circadian rhythm. When you travel to a different time zone, you should do the same. Don't use too much melatonin because you may have nightmares.

In summary, you will live longer and healthier if you enjoy eight hour of deep, refreshing sleep at night. You will look also younger as you reach your seventies and eighties. The key is reaching deep, refreshing sleep, or delta sleep, every night. If you are having problems with insomnia, I recommend making a list and reviewing what you are doing wrong to determine what to do to regain normal sleep and restore your normal circadian rhythm.

It is important to remember that you can't change your biology and circadian rhythms, which have developed over millions of years. Your body is already set to function as expected. Forcing your sleep system to do what you want may eventually lead to mental and physical problems. People who work graveyards or late at night may get away with it for a few weeks or months, but eventually they will pay a price with their health. No wonder so many people are having problems with sleep at night.

Our brain has adapted to the change of daylight to let us know it is time to go to sleep. With the discovery of electricity, humans have deceived the brain to create an altered reality and confusion. This is what troubles many individuals with insomnia. Their brains are in a state of confusion and feel disconnected with their internal regulatory hormonal systems. Their brains are constantly searching and pleading to return to the evolutionary circadian rhythm to reestablish balance and order to a system that has worked for millions of years to help the entire body to recover, continue to survive, and thrive. It is clear that the introduction of more light, alcohol, refined sugars, and toxic substances to our bodies has not helped to make our bodies healthier but has increased our levels of stress and the disorganization of many of our internal neurological and hormonal systems.

CHAPTER 7

S is for Sexuality

Sexual activity is a natural and physiological function of any human being. There is nothing dirty, sinful, or abnormal about our sex organs or their physiological functions. For centuries, sex was a taboo or a dirty word, equated with sin. Men and women were embarrassed or ostracized if they talked about their sex organs or behavior.

Men were encouraged by ancient cultures to dominate women and impose their sexuality upon them without regards to the women's feelings. Unfortunately, this kind of thinking still prevails in some cultures and civilized societies. Gradually, this kind of dominant behavior has been changing. In fact, the greatest advances in human sexuality have taken place in the last century. This progress has paralleled the advancement of the rights of women and their liberation from the oppressive behavior by male-dominated societies. This repression will eventually subside, and total equality of the sexes will be the norm.

In this book, I emphasized the ultimate goal for supreme happiness. Partners in search of long and healthy relationship should pursue love and happiness as their ultimate goal for a totally fulfilling relationship. When I started this book, my formula was simply DRESS. Then, it occurred to me that something was missing in achieving a healthy, fulfilling, and happy lifestyle. Sexuality and spirituality were missing from my original formula to complete the picture. The final letters in the amended formula (DRESS-SS) represent these two components, which I discuss in this chapter and the next.

As humans, we cannot deny the existence of our sexual organs and the hormones influencing our behaviors and the reactions of this normal function. Love is an emotional need. If you feel loved by your partner, you feel secure when he or she is present. The love of our partners enhances our sense of self-worth. Love is the basis for a more significant relationship. Love provides meaning and purpose. Sex is more enjoyable when you feel loved by someone who has your best interests in mind. When partners are committed to love and happiness, sex is like a wonderful dessert that helps us experience a life of greater happiness. This is what I emphasize in this chapter to help you reach optimal emotional health through sexuality. Stressful relationships sap you mood, motivation, and happiness. Sometimes it is better to stay single to be free of stress. If you are not involved in a relationship, you can still have orgasms by yourself to relieve tension and cortisol overdrive. You don't have to be committed to maintain your sex drive with someone else to keep you sexual drive going.

In chapter 2, "D is for Diet," I described how foods help to nourish our bodies to grow strong, healthy, and happy. The reality is that foods alone are not sufficient to reach greater happiness. The secret to happiness is a sense of attraction to the things that make us whole. We should become aware of the energy surrounding us and the energy coming from within us. We are not just physical beings but a composition of emotional, cognitive, and spiritual beings. Sexuality provides another avenue to reach our destination of happiness. When our sexual life is in tatters, we are unhappy, and negative thinking dominates our thoughts. When something goes wrong, people often react with anger, hate, jealousy, and despair, as if these negative feelings could bring back what has been lost. In the face of adversity, it is better to become aware of our feelings and channel our energy in a positive direction. Be resilient.

Love provides the guide to resolve conflicts. Negative feelings like hate and anger deprive the individual from attaining optimal love and happiness. Celibates may claim to be happy emotionally and spiritually when they suppress sexuality for a greater cause. This may be true when love is sublimated to a higher cause for spiritual reasons. However, the majority of individuals choose to find someone to love. It helps them feel significant and gives purpose to life. Sex is a natural and important experience in achieving happiness when love is the common bond between partners. It is up to us to enhance the joy of our sexuality and use this natural pleasure to reach greater happiness.

When two loving souls unite to obtain ultimate pleasure through sexual interaction, they experience one of the greatest joys of life. Unfortunately, for centuries, millions of men and women have grown unhappy and unfulfilled because of misunderstandings, taboos, misconceptions, and wrong interpretations of a natural physiological function available to us to enjoy a happier existence. Sadly, this prevents many partners from finding joy through sexual activity to reach ultimate happiness and often leads to the deterioration of relationships.

These false expectations and emotions can be the result of internal or external factors. Internal factors may come from emotions or negative feelings, such as anger, jealousy, and hate. Health problems and internal hormonal or chemical imbalances may play a role as well. External factors very often play a significant role. They may come in the form of financial troubles, religious issues, strained family relationships, political biases, or societal and cultural rules.

Authoritarian societies and cultures that treat sexual activity and sexual freedom as promiscuity impose high levels of anxiety and unnecessary suffering for no reason. Family members may interfere in a relationship of a couple, depriving them unfairly of achieving ultimate happiness. For centuries, religion has been very authoritarian and oppressive by classifying sex as a sinful activity. This was a totalitarian concept promoted by individuals deprived of sexual pleasures as a source of ultimate happiness.

In spite of greater advances, many societies and cultures still make laws to punish individuals who are in a loving relationship and want to make love the basis for their sexual attraction in their search for greater happiness. Of course, some norms and rules of common decency are necessary, but loving relationships should not be considered harmful if no damage is done to anyone. Protecting underage children from abuse and exploitation is still a responsibility of society so that children can fulfill their potential of ultimate happiness as adults. It is still society's responsibility to protect communities from sexually transmitted diseases. Infecting anyone with a virus or bacteria is, in reality, a crime that destroys the right of anyone to be happy and enjoy a healthy lifestyle. Protections from sexual predators and violence against any person are necessary since these individuals take away the happiness of innocent individuals.

Sex drive, unfortunately, changes over time. These changes take place because we produce less sex hormone as we age. In a previous chapter, I explained that, to bring our bodies in balance, we need to check our hormone levels from time to time to find out our deficiencies. Estrogen and testosterone levels decline over time, as do other hormones, which in turn affects the function of many cells. In men, a significant decline of testosterone leads to erectile dysfunction (ED). In women, low estrogen and testosterone levels decrease sexual drive and lead to physical symptoms like hot flashes, low levels of energy, irregular menstruation, and many adverse body changes.

Performance anxiety develops in men and may become an issue as men see the loss of strong erections as they age. The good news is that, with proper care and management of these imbalances, partners can enjoy great sex in their sixties, seventies, and beyond. As partners mature, they can enjoy a more pleasurable and satisfying sex life for many reasons. They include:

- A greater capacity to communicate and express love and intimacy
- Improved memory with increased sex
- A greater level of confidence in each other and no fears of rejection
- A greater satisfaction to enjoy a conversation with others about love and sexual satisfaction without inhibitions
- A greater interest in making life more meaningful and full of purpose
- A greater sense of gratitude for the life they have enjoyed together
- A greater interest in a healthier lifestyle, including adopting healthy diets to prevent illness
- A feeling of wellness by exercising more to stay in shape and look attractive to each other
- A greater sense of realism of what love means and what is important as life continues to fade

Can a couple enjoy great sex after Fifty?

There is no reason not to enjoy great sex after fifty and beyond. A couple should visit their doctor for yearly checkups. A medical evaluation should include testing for sex hormone levels (estrogens and testosterone), thyroid levels, sugar and cholesterol levels, vitamin D levels, magnesium, and a complete blood count (CBC) at a minimum. Men should ask for a PSA level to detect possible prostate cancer before taking testosterone. The same is true for women. They should have mammograms if there is a history of cancer of the breast in the family or there is a suspicious mass in the breast. Estrogen replacement may not be possible if there is genetic evidence of cancer in the family or cancer in the breast. However, even in the presence of cancer, a couple can maintain a healthy sexual relationship based on love and mutual understanding of their limitations. Love is the main ingredient in a healthy and loving relationship.

Telomere testing to assess your genes and longevity is a useful test to guide you to determine whether you need to make changes to prolong life and health. Different laboratories in the United States offer this test through the mail for under $100. (See the resources section at the end of this book.)

My recommendation for many couples as they age is to reject all the myths that there is no sexual life as we age. A couple should adapt and make adjustments to body changes, accept new ways to approach such changes, and make an investment if necessary to improve the body and health. Recent studies in Canada and Australia demonstrate improvements in short-term memory with increased sex in couples over fifty years of age. Women and men shouldn't hesitate making themselves more attractive. Some may opt for cosmetic surgery, breast implants, fillers, Botox, supplements, and workouts. Any change to make you look and feel better is acceptable. You are entitled to do whatever makes you and your partner look happier. Why not do it if it makes you look younger and feel better?

Can estrogens, progesterone, and testosterone help women to stay younger and healthy after menopause?

If there is no evidence or family history of cancer of the ovaries and or breast, a woman should consider estrogen replacement therapy during menopause. Even in the even that a woman carries the BRCA1 and 2 genes associated with breast and ovarian cancer, there is a solution. Today, many women can have their breasts removed and replaced by an implant to prevent breast cancer. The same is true for the ovaries. If they have no children yet, they can have the eggs removed to be fertilized and maintained in a frozen state until they are ready to have children through a surrogate mother. Women who have had their breasts, Fallopian tubes, and ovaries removed can become potential candidates for hormone replacement therapy.

Estrogen is a hormone that affects all cells of the body. Most cells have estrogen receptors for their physiological functions and overall wellness. Without estrogen, the body experiences many changes. Women begin to notice their hair is not as shiny or the texture is changing. Some women feel they are losing their hair. Their nails break more often; the skin begins to wrinkle or sag, the breasts begin to drop, and the energy levels decrease. Some women experience hot flashes and night sweats, which become more intense as they enter menopause. Women may also develop insomnia and feel tired even at the start of the day. Eventually, bones become weaker due to osteopenia and osteoporosis, leading to compression fractures in the spine and loss of height. Some women develop compression fractures of the spine and humps known as kyphosis. Women who do not take estrogen after menopause age faster than women who remain in estrogen therapy years after menopause.

Estriol is an effective treatment for relieving menopausal symptoms. A six-month study of fifty-two women with severe symptomatology found that supplementation with 2 to 8 mg of estriol succinate produced significant improvements within one month, which continued throughout the therapy. Estriol also reversed vaginal atrophy and improved the quality of cervical mucus. Vaginal creams and other bio-identical hormones prepared by a compound pharmacy are more effective as well. Bio-identical estrogen and progesterone are more effective than synthetic forms of these hormones. Look for a doctor who prescribes bio-identical hormones. These hormones and creams are prepared by qualified compound pharmacies. My wife uses a bio-identical estrogen vaginal cream, which is very effective.

In addition to estrogen, women need to check their testosterone levels. Testosterone in small amounts provides women with increased libido and sexual enjoyment. Testosterone is the hormone of desire. Testosterone levels normally peak at the time of ovulation, when a woman is more fertile. The rise of testosterone midway through the cycle stimulates the desire in women for sex. The ovaries produce about one-quarter of the testosterone in women. If a woman has a total hysterectomy with removal of the ovaries, she loses about one-quarter of her testosterone.

According to the Mayo Clinic, if you haven't had your uterus removed, your doctor will typically prescribe estrogen, along with progesterone or progestin (progesterone-like medication). This is because estrogen alone, when not balanced by progesterone, can stimulate growth of the lining of the uterus, increasing the risk of uterine cancer. If you have had your uterus removed (hysterectomy), you don't need to take progestin.

In the largest clinical trial to date, a combination estrogen-progestin pill (Prempro) increased the risk of certain serious conditions, including:

Heart disease
Stroke
Blood clots
Breast cancer

Subsequent studies have suggested that these risks vary depending on age. For example, women who begin hormone therapy more than ten or twenty years from the onset of menopause or at age sixty or older are at greater risk of the above conditions. But if hormone therapy is started before the age of sixty or within ten years of menopause, the benefits appear to outweigh the risks.

The risks of hormone therapy may also vary depending on whether estrogen is given alone or with progestin, the dose and type of estrogen, and other health factors, such as your risks of heart and blood vessel (cardiovascular) disease, cancer risks, and family medical history.

All of these risks should be considered in deciding whether hormone therapy might be an option for you.

Despite its health risks, systemic bio-identical estrogen is still the most effective treatment for menopausal symptoms. The benefits of hormone therapy may outweigh the risks if you're healthy and you:

- Experience moderate to severe hot flashes or other menopausal symptoms
- Have lost bone mass and either can't tolerate or aren't benefiting from other treatments
- Stopped having periods before age forty (premature menopause) or lost normal function of your ovaries before age forty (premature ovarian insufficiency)

Women who experience early menopause, particularly those who've had their ovaries removed and don't take estrogen therapy until at least age forty-five, have a higher risk of:

Osteoporosis
Heart disease
Earlier death
Parkinson's-like symptoms (parkinsonism)
Anxiety or depression

For women who reach menopause prematurely, the protective benefits of hormone therapy usually outweigh the risks.

Your age, type of menopause, and time since menopause play significant roles in the risks associated with hormone therapy. Talk with your doctor about your personal risks.

About one-quarter of testosterone is produced in the ovary, a quarter is produced in the adrenal gland, and one-half is produced from various precursors produced in the ovaries and adrenal gland. There is also much interconversion among steroid hormones. The main precursor in the ovary is androstenedione, which is converted primarily to estrone, but which can also be converted to androgens. The main precursors in the adrenal gland are DHEA and DHEA-S (Guay 2002) If a woman is taking estrogens only, the estrogen is the dominant hormone, which in turn decreases the circulating small amount of free testosterone. Women typically experience low libido after the removal of their ovaries. The solution to this problem is testosterone supplementation until they reach levels similar to young women with normal ovaries. Testosterone, in addition to increasing desire and libido, improves vaginal and bladder tone, decreases body fat, improves muscle strength and bone density, enhances function of thyroid hormone, relieves anxiety and depression, and improves cognitive function. If the testosterone levels in a woman are low, she should take testosterone sublingually or use a testosterone cream. A woman who has had a hysterectomy should have her testosterone levels checked frequently to get to the right dose.

Testosterone and effects on a man

Testosterone is a sex hormone made in the testicles and adrenal glands. If testosterone helps women's desire, imagine what it can do for millions of men with low testosterone levels. This hormone is what distinguishes boys from men. As boys mature, their voices change to bass; facial hair grows in abundance; muscles develop; strength increases; thoughts of the opposite sex increase; and erections increase in frequency, along with an increase in sexual desire. Testosterone is what gives men powerful muscles and strength, sex drive, and sperm production. Testosterone helps to keep bones strong and build muscle mass.

Testosterone levels can drop as a man ages. This decline is usually apparent in men after age fifty. Low testosterone makes erections soft and results in loss of sexual drive, a condition known as erectile dysfunction (ED). In some men, this could be congenital. Hypogonadism is a condition in which a person is born with low testosterone. Hypogonadism is also a condition when testosterone levels fall below normal levels, even in men who were normal before.

Low testosterone can affect a man's sex life, mood, and sexual activity significantly. It can also affect his overall health. Obesity, diabetes, and possible heart disease have been linked to low testosterone levels. Fortunately, doctors can treat low testosterone levels. It requires an evaluation by a doctor and blood work to check the levels of total and free testosterone. Treatment may improve a man's erections, sex drive, muscle mass, sleep, energy level, and mood. A man with total testosterone levels below 260 mg/dL needs testosterone supplementation. Dosage should be titrated until levels are between 500 to 900 mg/dL. It is important to use a dosage that helps the symptoms, not the lab value.

Before taking testosterone, a PSA test is necessary to check that there is no evidence of cancer of the prostate. If the PSA is elevated, a man may need a biopsy. If the biopsy is negative, he can be treated with testosterone. There are testosterone lotions and creams, but the most effective way to raise testosterone levels is through injections of 100 to 200 mg of testosterone cypionate. An intramuscular injection once a week may be necessary. A new blood level check is required after four weeks. At that time, the dosage could be changed to 100 to 200 mg every two weeks thereafter. Injections can be used in combination with HCG (human chorionic gonadotropin), 250 IU subcutaneously, two days before the testosterone injection to maintain the hypothalamus testicular axis feedback mechanism active.

A doctor should check the testosterone levels every three to six months to determine the effective dose. In addition, a complete blood count is necessary to check for increased hemoglobin levels, which may cause polycythemia. Only a doctor qualified to treat these problems can determine the optimal dose of testosterone.

In addition to testosterone, a man can use Viagra or Cialis to improve his erections. Pumps and rings can help to increase the hardness of the penis in cases not responding to hormones and Viagra or Cialis. Furthermore, diets rich in L-arginine and L-citrulline help to increase the blood flow in the pelvic organs. These foods increase vasodilation, which in turn improves erections. Rings are also useful to maintain erections and improve ED.

DHEA Supplementation

Dehydroepiandrosterone, or DHEA, is a hormone that declines during the aging process. The adrenal gland and brain produce DHEA in women and men. Blood levels begin to drop around the age of thirty, and men and women begin to have a deficiency of this vital hormone by the age of forty. The rate of decline continues at a rate of 1 percent per year. By age sixty, a man or a woman may have a declined level of DHEA of greater than 50 percent. Many men and women over fifty have very low levels of DHEA. To balance deficiencies through supplementation, blood testing is essential. Deficiencies of DHEA have been correlated with numerous age-related conditions, including chronic inflammation, immune dysfunction, depression, rheumatoid arthritis, increased risk for certain cancers, excess body fat, cognitive decline, osteoporosis, and some complications of type 2 diabetes. Women with a history of breast or ovarian cancer should not use DHEA as a supplement, since the body converts this hormone to estrogen.

If blood levels are low, I recommend starting with 25 mg a day of DHEA for two weeks. If no side effects exist and tolerance is good, I usually raise the dosage to 50 mg per day. To find out if the dosage is effective, a new blood level is required. A level from 350 to 430 mcg/dL is optimal. Because DHEA does not follow the menstrual cycle, doctors can prescribe it on a daily basis.

Scientific studies have shown that a dose of 50 mg of DHEA in women improves physical and psychological well-being by 84 percent. Balancing hormone deficiencies helps bring hormonal function to a normal equilibrium for better health. A normal hormonal function helps to strengthen the immune system as well.

CHAPTER 8

S is for Spirituality

Is spirituality connected to health?

We are connected in a spiritual way to all other life forms. We find in trees, plants, and flowers a spiritual interconnection. We love the beauty of an old oak tree and would do whatever it takes to protect it. Plants affect us the same way; we love the colors and fragrances of flowers. They project beauty, serenity, and peace. There is no question that we feel a connection with our environment. We even feel sorrow if a beautiful tree or plant dies. We also feel interconnected to our animals, domestic and wild. We wonder how they—and even we—have survived for millions of years. We depend on them for our needs and survival. Many herbs have healing qualities, and many drugs are based on the discovery of the plants' healing qualities. Currently, we can find hundreds—if not thousands—of herbs with healing properties, which we use as supplements to our diets. We feel there is a spiritual connection that goes beyond ourselves. When we look at the universe, we find an equilibrium that is difficult to explain because of our imperfections.

Why is there such order and balance in the universe or within our own bodies? If we use an analysis, we can compare our bodies to a universe of galaxies and stars populated by different communities with their own rules, missions, and functions that are all interconnected in spite of their differences. Metaphorically, the "liver galaxy" makes proteins and processes nutritional elements and delivers them to all the other "galaxies" of the body (brain, lungs, and so on). When something goes wrong in one star or galaxy, this interconnection becomes more obvious. A mutant cell anywhere may begin to affect the others and invade neighbors, causing great damage and destruction and threatening the entire universe. In desperation, all organs appeal to a greater force to find a solution to a problem beyond themselves, thereby threatening the survival of all these communities and the entire universe. Their desperate voices finally reach the intellect, a superior force inside us that oversees and determines the best solution for this desperate problem, and hope is on the way.

When our intellect makes a conscious decision that something is wrong, we look for help to find the cure and stop the proliferating cancer cells from destroying their neighbors and threatening the existence or our entire universe. This demonstrates the power of our mind-body connection. However, when we realize that a problem is beyond our power to control, even with professional and technological help, we look beyond our universe. That is when our minds look to our creator for help.

What is spirituality?

For many cultures and religions, spirituality is a belief in a higher power or a force operating in the universe. This force provides interconnection with all living creatures, offers purpose and meaning to life, and develops personal values. Through spirituality, people find meaning, hope, comfort, inner peace, and protection.

Spirituality is also associated with music, art, and beautiful creations, in addition to religion. Beautiful creations fascinate us, as do inspired men and women like Michelangelo, the famous painter and sculptor; Mozart; Robert and Clara Schumann, composers and pianists; and many others who produce works superior to other artists. We see the hand of God in their works to help explain the beauty and meaning of their work. Spirituality moves people to be compassionate, selfless, charitable, supportive, and loving. Spirituality promotes the good in us to minimize our inner negative feelings and tendencies.

Spirituality aids our health by relieving stress and helping those with anxiety and depression through coping skills, hope, and inner peace. Because it relieves stress, spirituality helps to prevent high levels of cortisol and adrenaline, which affect our hormonal and immune systems. In chapter 5, which focuses on stress, I explained how stress can downgrade our immune system, making us more susceptible to infection or cancer. Spirituality helps our bodies to have a strong immune system to protect us against bacteria, viruses, and many other illnesses. Spirituality also helps those who are addicted to drugs or alcohol or who possess a violent character. Spirituality helps us to develop humility in order to improve relationships with our spouses, children, siblings, family, friends, and even our enemies.

Spirituality provides comfort in desperate situations or tragedies. The first action at our personal or community level is to pray and ask God, as a supreme force of good, to help us to cope and get over a difficult injury or tragedy. Spirituality serves as a permanent healer and helps us to learn how to forgive and forget. By forgiving someone who has hurt us or caused great injury to our families, we learn to move beyond the pain and stress that the injury has caused to our emotional and intellectual well-being. Forgiveness diminishes stress, anxiety, anger, insomnia, depression, and feelings of hopelessness. Above all, spirituality promotes love and a feeling of happiness. In *Living Longer and Reversing Aging*, I emphasized from the beginning the need to pursue, as our ultimate goal in life, love and happiness. Spirituality provides the guide and the structure to achieve this goal.

As a personal note, I will tell the story of Bill, my lawyer, patient, and friend, which is a story about the most incredible power of mind over body, spirituality, and faith. When Bill passed away, I gave his eulogy to emphasize his capacity to recover from illness in an almost miraculous way. Bill had had a heart transplant twenty years earlier and enjoyed relatively good health, even though he had to take medication to prevent rejection of the heart transplant.

One day, while he was in the hospital, Bill asked me to visit him at the hospital and offer an opinion about his doctor's recommendation to amputate his leg, which was cyanotic due to a blood clot. When I saw his foot, the skin was very dark, and I felt there was no hope but to amputate. Before giving him my opinion, I felt it was prudent to ask for another opinion from a vascular surgeon. The surgeon suggested a trial with anticoagulants for another week. After eight days of anticoagulant therapy, the foot began to change color and eventually became pink. He never had to face amputation or any other procedure. Bill told me later he had a weapon to fight the clot; it was prayer.

Bill was a very spiritual man and had a deep and profound faith in God. Before his heart transplant, Bill told me he was at peace with himself and felt that it was in God's hands if he was allowed to survive. He had no fear of dying or having his old aching heart removed from his chest. The same thing happened when the doctor told him that his leg had to be amputated. He had faith in God that he would recover and be able to keep his leg.

The second incredible episode occurred one day after Bill attended an opera in Houston. He became very ill that night. Within hours, he went into a coma. His diagnosis was septicemia secondary to ruptured diverticula in the colon. Before falling into a coma, he prayed. A few days later, after surgery and antibiotic therapy, he said he was feeling well and wanted to go to his church to teach Sunday school. He eventually went home and enjoyed a relatively good life for many years despite his age. I was amazed by his faith following his recovery.

Years later after he died, I was asked by his wife to give the eulogy at his church. He was a popular lawyer and well loved by his community.

In the eulogy, I emphasized the power of the mind over the body and the power of spirituality. After the service, his pastor told me it was Bill's faith in God that kept him alive when he was very ill and close to death. He said that his community prayed with and for him, and Bill stayed in touch with his pastor all the time.

I will never forget Bill. He is the clearest example of how mind over body, coupled with an extraordinary faith in God, can help a person through extraordinarily difficult circumstances.

Bill's faith in God inspired me to add this chapter to my basic longevity DRESS-SS code. I realized I could not leave spirituality and faith aside. It is important to me as a doctor and a healer to offer spirituality to my patients and readers. This important tool can help with decisions that will lead to peace within our minds and bodies. Faith in God is a powerful healing tool to have available when confronting difficult choices and decisions about health or death.

How can spirituality help us to reach happiness as we age?

Like it or not, we will age. Our bodies will begin to experience a decline after age thirty. Many of the changes are very subtle and become more apparent over time. Spirituality, like emotional and intellectual development, grows over time. We grow physically, intellectually, emotionally, and spiritually during our life spans. We are, in fact, the union of four beings to become whole. Each being grows at a different pace depending on our environment, personal experiences, and education. Some people may stop growing emotionally, intellectually, or physically at one point their lives.

Some people with emotional problems may have slowed their growth in the emotional sphere at a very early age, depending on environmental circumstances. Poverty, lack of love, or a bad family may have slowed down the growth of their emotional being. Painful memories of emotional injuries may have caused significant trauma and difficulty trusting others or accepting love. This lack of love may become the missing ingredient affecting many people suffering from persistent anxiety or stress. No wonder those suffering from this deficiency have more difficulties making friends or having a successful marriage.

Some people may have grown intellectually and become geniuses in their fields of training but lack the emotional growth to deal with others or to project or provide love and compassion. It is not uncommon to see these intellectuals acting impulsively and without compassion. Some become delusional neurotics who constantly reject reality. Despotic dictators are good examples of such individuals. They destroy lives and torture their opponents.

Most likely, those without emotional growth reject spirituality. Their egos and negative thinking rejects goodness and compassion. Any expression of spirituality is feeble or nonexistent. They are weak, emotionally and spiritually.

In our daily lives, there are people who behave the same. A despotic boss, teacher, husband, father, or politician can act similarly, causing deep pain and scars that may last a long time and have serious consequences. Those affected may become dependent on medications to relieve anxiety, depression, or pain. Some become addicted to opioids, which contributes to destroying them and their families.

Growing spiritually helps to balance an uncontrolled emotional being full of hatred, envy, jealousy, rage, depression, anxiety, and negativity, leading to drug dependency.

Spirituality and healing

Ayurveda emerged from Vedic literature, based on spirituality, more than five thousand years ago in India. Early practitioners sought to achieve a state of balance and health in the mind and body and to reach a creative union with a creative source or God. This unified relationship of religion and medicine existed for thousands of years until recently, with the growth of scientific medicine in the Western world.

Jesus and many religious figures were known for their remarkable healing powers and abilities as much as their spiritual guidance and direction.

When there were no effective medicines, prayer was the only way to cope with a serious illness or infection. Many physicians, however, have lost the spiritual guidance they gave to their patients a few decades ago. Most of them have become believers of the scientific method and discarded spirituality. The losers are their patients, unless they take the initiative with their families and pastors to find comfort for their suffering in spirituality and prayer.

Several studies have demonstrated the positive influence of spirituality, prayer, and meditation on longevity.

In 2012 in the journal *ISRN Psychiatry*, a study showed that spiritual practices are associated with many health benefits. This study reviewed thousands of studies published from 1872 to 2010. The researchers found that about 80 percent of the studies involved mental health problems. The study found that those who are spiritual are usually more positive, optimistic, and have a better sense of purpose in life and improved self-esteem. They are usually happier than those who are not spiritual. They also enjoy life more, in spite of their pain, and suffer less from depression and anxiety or drug dependency. Many other studies have found that spirituality helps to enhance recovery from illness and surgery. It also helps those dealing with grief and death of a loved one. As a bonus, many people who are spiritual tend not to smoke cigarettes or engage in risky sexual behaviors. Spirituality promotes healthy behaviors and helps to reduce complications from common diseases.

Physicians shouldn't ignore all these benefits derived from spiritual practices. They should help to promote and encourage their patients to speak to their pastors or preachers for comfort and spiritual guidance.

I am a believer in spirituality as an assistant to medical treatment. The story of my friend Bill was an opportunity to see spirituality in action; it was, for me, an enlightening experience. Spirituality helps to guide our actions to make life-and-death decisions. As a doctor, I also value spirituality in medical decisions. It is my practice to encourage my patients to pray and search for spiritual guidance. It works.

As we age, we grow in maturity and wisdom as selfishness declines, and we begin to understand others. Compassion also grows and becomes enhanced when we face pain and loss and learn how to deal with suffering.

CHAPTER 9

Genetic and Telomere Research on Longevity and DNA

We are getting closer to reverse aging

Researchers are getting closer every day to reversing aging and extending our longevity.

At the University of Texas in San Antonio, scientists are conducting research in a mouse that is living longer than its peers. MouseUT25298 looks younger and stronger than other mice of the same age. This special mouse is being fed with an antibiotic known as rapamycin used to prevent organ rejection after transplantation (Park and O'Connor 2015, 10–15). Rapamycin appears to delay aging in mice of any age, suggesting that aging can be delayed in people of any age as well. The way this antibiotic works is by interrupting the function of a gene named mTOR, present in mice and human beings. This gene appears to affect how energy is used by the cell, depending on the caloric intake. The gene becomes very active when plenty of food or nutrients are available and becomes quiet when caloric intake is restricted. This finding suggests that, when caloric intake is restricted, the cells are not overwhelmed by the amount of nutrients to be processed and the exposure to free radicals that damage the DNA from the oxidative process when the cell is active most of the time.

Other promising research in this field is worth mentioning. One is the study of the telomeres. Telomeres are the endings of the chromosomes that can become short or long depending on the activity of an enzyme, telomerase. When telomeres become short, their life span is shortened. When the telomeres are long, the life span of the cell is extended. Extending the life of the telomeres by activating telomerase reverses aging and prevents premature death of the cell. Keeping the telomeres long also helps to prevent age-related diseases, which ultimately reverses aging.

Elizabeth Blackburn, PhD, and winner of the Nobel Prize in Medicine in 2009, with coauthor Elissa Epel, PhD, explain how behaviors, food, and the environment can shorten telomeres in *The Telomere Effect: A Revolutionary Approach to Living Younger, Healthier, Longer* (Blackburn and Epel 2016) In another study, Amy Wagers of Harvard Stem Cell Institute, found that GDF11, a protein present in young animals, when given to older animals, rejuvenates tissues and improves function. Neurobiologist Dena Dubai is investigating Klotho, a newly discovered hormone found in animals that appears to increase longevity by 30 percent. About one in five people also carries a version of the Klotho gene that boosts its amounts. On average, those people live an extra three to four years. It is not the hormone of immortality, but it's a start (Park and O'Connor 2015, 10–15).

All of these are promising areas of research into reversing aging and prolonging longevity. If we can eliminate many chronic illnesses, dying from age-related illnesses may become something of the past. Scientists are currently extending life in their labs and are very optimistic. What is important is extending the quality of life to make people healthier as they age.

In 2013, Professor Dongcheng Cai of Albert Einstein College of Medicine in Philadelphia found that stem cells in the hypothalamus decrease as we age, and the decline accelerates aging but is reversible when these cells are replenished. By injecting hypothalamic stem cells in the brains of mice with loss of cells, researchers were able to reverse aging. It appears these stem cells produce a molecule called microRNA. When these molecules are released into the cerebrospinal fluid, it reverses the aging process. It is now possible to do embryonic genetic editing to repair serious mutations resulting in severe genetic illnesses. In the future, scientists could eliminate many degenerative diseases and many inherited diseases from mutations with genetic engineering. For example, women with the BRCA gene that causes cancer of the breast and ovaries could have their embryos edited at the time of fertilization to eliminate this cancer in their daughters. By eliminating degenerative diseases, it will be possible for future generations to prolong their longevity by decades, even centuries.

What are some examples of using genetic information in the treatment of disease?

A person's genetic makeup affects how his or her body breaks down certain medicines. Genetic testing can examine certain liver enzymes in a person to find out how his or her body breaks down and removes medicines from the body. Because these liver enzymes are less active in some people, they are less able to break down and get rid of some medicines. This can lead to serious side effects. This type of testing is being used to find the right dose of certain medicines, such as antidepressants that are used to treat some mental illnesses.

There is now a test to find out whether a medicine called Herceptin will be an effective treatment in breast cancer. This test looks at "estrogen receptors" in tumors.

Children with a common type of childhood leukemia can be tested to find the right doses of chemotherapy treatment. Genetic sequencing for precision treatment with the right medicine is the future of cancer treatment. People with cancer can expect to increase their longevity with new treatments already available or under investigation. Defeating cancer will allow people to live longer and enjoy a better future. Cancer survivors want to live healthier lives and enjoy every moment after their dreadful experience. They have a greater appreciation for life and happiness.

Can we prevent genes from expressing themselves to prevent illness?

Medicine and nutrition are advancing at a rapid pace, and the day to find the causes of many chronic illnesses, including cancer, is not far away. By controlling your environment, you can prevent many illnesses that shorten your life span. If you follow my prescription or code, you can delay or prevent a bad gene from expressing or developing a defect that may lead to illnesses like diabetes, heart disease, arthritis, dementia, mental illness, or cancer.

Clara, my wife, contributed to this book by practicing what we believe. She is an avid reader of nutrition books and knows how to prepare healthy meals and to create a lifestyle and an environment of love and happiness. She is disciplined with her diet. We have been married over fifty years, and during that time, she eliminated substantially all sugars, syrups, and starches from our diet. We eat a well-balanced diet that is rich in vegetables, fruits, nuts, fish, fiber, and some supplements. Her motivation was the presence of diabetes in her parents, grandparents, relatives, and siblings. Her decision to do something, because of this genetic inheritance, to prevent these genes from expressing themselves is the main reason she has kept the same weight she had when we got married and continues to look younger and healthier than others with her chronological age. You can appreciate this in the pictures in this book. As a result, she is the only person in her family who has remained diabetes free.

I tell this story to emphasize the point that we can modify our environment to prevent illnesses, in spite of our genetic inheritance or predisposition to any illness. I personally have learned a lot from reading the many articles and books that she has screened for me. I also value her advice, ideas, and assistance in researching countless journals and magazines. My own personal experience as a doctor who has spent a lifetime reading medical journals, books, magazines, newspapers, and searching the internet has helped me to develop concepts about aging and living healthier. My patients and, I hope, all readers can become the beneficiaries of our personal experience and my fifty years of medical practice.

As a medical doctor, I was privileged to work in my early years of practice with doctors who pioneered treatments in the fields of nutrition and heart surgery. In the late 1960s, as a young resident at the University of Pennsylvania hospital in Philadelphia, I met a young surgeon, Stanley J. Dudrick, MD. Years later, he became a widely recognized pioneer in the development of the specialized central venous feeding technique known as intravenous hyperalimentation (IVH) or total parenteral nutrition (TPN). The medical community recognizes his development and subsequent successful clinical application of this highly effective therapeutic modality as one of the four most significant accomplishments in the history of the development of modern surgery, together with the discovery and development of asepsis and antisepsis, antibiotic therapy, and anesthesia (*JAMA* 239 1978, 192). His work is acknowledged as one of the three most important advancements in surgery during the past century, along with open-heart surgery and organ transplantation.

I also had the opportunity to work with Denton Cooley, MD, the renowned heart surgeon in Houston who pioneered the first artificial heart transplants. Through a collaborative effort, we developed nutritional and exercise programs for people recovering from heart surgery in the 1980s. We also developed advanced cardiac rehabilitation programs and evaluations for elite athletes to maximize their biological functions. Ever since, I have incorporated in my practice programs to improve nutrition for the prevention of heart disease and other illnesses. Years of practicing these principles led me to summarize this experience in an easy to remember code, DRESS-SS. By following my code or prescription, you can enjoy a healthier lifestyle, live longer, delay or reverse aging, and prevent illnesses despite a defective genetic code.

Following my prescription requires self-discipline and changes in behavior for successful outcomes. This longevity code, or prescription, may help you to get closer to the elusive fountain of youth millions of people before you have dreamed of finding. My prescription, if it is followed faithfully, will help you to reach your final destination of health and happiness. You can expect to reach your final days on this planet in the best possible physical, emotional, intellectual, and spiritual shape. In this book, I offer information about how to keep all your hormones, chemistries, and enzymatic activity of cells in check and to alert you of any imbalances or deficiencies. Keeping the body in balance throughout your life span will help you find the perfect equilibrium of health to keep illness away.

Your job is to make all cells function as well-oiled machines, capable of responding to any injuries or any unexpected event for faster recovery. Biologically, our bodies require a well-balanced neural-hormonal-immune system complex for optimal wellness. Keeping all the chemicals involved in the neurotransmission of nerve impulses and hormones that affect almost all cells in your body in perfect balance will aid the immune system to be prepared to defend your body against powerful enemies from the outside, as well as the inside when your cells or tissues decide to go against you. If your immune system remains in top shape, you can prevent viruses or bacteria from making you sick and fight off cancer and other diseases. Today, we know, it is possible to kill cancer cells with our own killer white cells through cancer immunotherapy. A strong defense system is the key to maintaining our complex neuroendocrine systems to function in harmony with our bodies.

The answers to fight many illnesses reside within our bodies. If we live a life of wellness and free of illness, we can expect to live longer, stay healthy, and biologically look younger. To do this, however, you have to live a lifestyle that promotes wellness. You also need to develop awareness and knowledge about how to live well and about what is best for you. You need to read books and magazines to know what is good or bad for you, what can kill you, and what you can do to prevent it. Those who practice a lifetime of learning will always be ahead of those who do not. They will use their skills and knowledge to find the foods, systems, and behaviors to change their environments to promote wellness, increase their longevity, and decrease the possibility of illnesses, injuries, deficiencies, and problems associated with premature aging. You must find and tap the reservoir of best health practices and defenses for healthier living. You can do this by balancing your needs and wants. It all begins with good nutrition, proper rest, exercise, good restful sleep, stress management, a healthy sex life, and a rich spiritual life.

Is wellness the answer for our well-being and happiness in the future?

The best doctor is the one who leads his or her patients toward a healthier lifestyle for optimal wellness through prevention of illness and a periodic assessment of deficiencies or changes that may affect health and longevity. This concept of wellness, if applied every day to the life of any individual can help to decrease the cost of medical care everywhere in the world. Individuals, families, communities, states, and nations that promote wellness and healthier lifestyles and communities may see their health expenses and budgets decrease. By practicing these changes, future generations can live better lives. Illnesses will be easily managed, chronic disease will be defeated, and pain and suffering will be prevented and diminished.

My wife and I have no doubts; a healthier lifestyle will lead to greater happiness and longevity. We hope this book can become your companion everywhere. Keep it with you if you want to live a healthy lifestyle and especially if you are in the process of making changes and adjustments such as losing weight, exercising to stay fit, working to reverse aging, preventing illness, or recovering from cancer or any serious illness. We recommend that governments, corporations, businesses, and schools take notice and use this book to educate people and children by advising them to adopt and use the practical advice and concepts it offers.

We are born with good or bad genes that we inherit from our parents. This genetic code determines our health and life span. However, in spite of defective genes that predispose us to different diseases, we can modify our behaviors, our diets, and our environments to prevent the expression of those diseases. All this is possible if we know what to do to change and alter our biology. Once our minds are made up, it is possible to prevent illness and minimize the effects of defective gene inheritance.

We do not have to live like our parents and grandparents. For centuries, they were not aware of their genetic inheritance and did not know what to do when they carried defective genes that predisposed them to many illnesses. Even in the event our grandparents knew, there were no ways to prevent illness. They did not have the scientific advances in medicine and nutrition that we enjoy today to delay or prevent the expression of defective genetic inheritance. Our awareness and knowledge are powerful tools to help us fight illness or defective genes. We are privileged to know that, by improving nutrition or making changes in our environment and behaviors, we can affect our genes, our telomeres, and the health of our cells to enjoy better health and longevity.

The good news is that we don't have to live with the consequences of the defective genetic code we inherited. Recent research demonstrates that we can modify our genetic codes through behaviors, proper nutrition, medicines, and genetic interventions to provide precision medicines thanks to modern scientific methods. In the future, doctors will correct serious illnesses or genetic defects through genetic interventions and use genetic sequencing to select the best nutrients or medicines and immunotherapy. Ideally, if we can prevent the gene from expressing a defect or illness through a change in our environment, behavior, or lifestyle, we should try this first. Most recent research demonstrates that changing our diet and environment can indeed lengthen our telomeres in our genes.

Dr. Michael Murray, in *The Magic of Food*, reports on how good nutrition lowers the risk of genetic disease expression. In a 2000 landmark study at Duke University, researchers found that fat mice with yellow furs carry the agouti gene, which made them fat and yellow. This gene increases dramatically their risk of developing cancer and diabetes. Before their offspring were conceived, a test group of mother mice was fed a diet rich in vitamin B12, folic acid, and SAM-e. The baby mice were born brown and slender and, as they matured, didn't succumb to cancer and diabetes. The nutritional intervention in the mothers had completely erased the cancerous, diabetic genetic destiny of the agouti mice. Although the brown mice had the same genome as the yellow mice, the expression of the genome was significantly different because of nutritional factors. This is another instance of the magic of food and proof that genetic tendencies can be changed with dietary and nutritional approaches.

As a young medical doctor, I became aware of how a toxic environment, poor behaviors, and bad nutrition were killing people much too early. As an intern working in the emergency room of a hospital in Philadelphia in the 1960s, I noticed that many of the patients arriving to the ER were not older than fifty and were dying of heart attacks. *Why are these men dying so young?* I wondered.

At the time, we did not know very much about diet or the causes of atherosclerosis or coronary artery disease. The field of cardiovascular surgery was in the early stages, and there were no medicines to prevent the formation of plaque in the arteries or formation of clots. Stent procedures did not exist. Any person with serious coronary disease was most likely to die within a short time, depending on the severity of the obstruction. Life span was limited for survivors, since there were not many medicines or procedures to prevent more damage or ways to relieve the obstruction of a coronary.

In another occasion during my internship, one day I was assigned to the cancer section of the hospital. On my first day, my job was to take the histories and perform the physical exams of all the patients coming that week for treatment. The number of patients I saw the first week with cancer appalled me. Over twenty patients admitted that week had lung cancer. All were smokers. Doctors admitted them for chemotherapy since lung resections were very dangerous and full of medical complications. I was glad then I was not a smoker. Early in my years in medical school, I had the feeling smoking was not good for your health. While working at that hospital, I had proof that smoking kills people before their time. I had identified another destructive behavior that shortens the life spans of so many people.

Fortunately, we have come a long way and learned a great deal. Today we have better medicines, advanced diagnostic procedures, and surgical interventions to treat the problems that killed so many people at a younger age not so long ago. All these advances are wonderful and welcome. However, the basic problem continues. People still smoke and eat foods that cause obesity and heart problems. Millions smoke and develop emphysema, lung cancer, and many other preventable diseases. Others continue to have extensive exposure to the sun and ultraviolet radiation, which leads to skin cancer and premature aging. Some of the people who develop these problems may not even have any genetic factors to develop such diseases.

They develop heart disease or cancer because of their behaviors, not because of their genetic code. They create a destructive and toxic environment of their own to damage their chromosomes, mitochondria, and nuclear DNA.

We know that a diet rich in bad fats, trans fats, and cholesterol can lead to coronary artery disease even in the absence of any genetic factor. The same thing happens with lung cancer when people are exposed to thousands of toxic chemicals in cigarette smoke or hours of ultraviolet radiation resulting in skin cancer. In these types of situations, there is no need to have a genetic factor for lung or skin cancer. Most of the damage done to our cells—and by extension to our bodies—is caused by our own behaviors and not by our genes.

Why do people behave in such reckless ways that result in harm to their bodies, pain and disability, and shortened life spans?

To answer this question, I always go back to basics. I feel that lack of information through deficient education deprives people of awareness to prevent harm to their bodies. Many neglect to use the power of their minds to protect the most precious possession—their bodies—from harm, bad behaviors, poor diets, stress, and a toxic environment. Improving this lack of awareness is a necessary skill to survive. A good education about our basic needs regarding how to feed ourselves and how to protect our bodies from harm by our environment should start early. These skills should begin in the schools when children are open to learning and acquiring skills for survival; this should be reinforced in the home and become a necessary skill throughout our life spans. Governments should make wellness education mandatory for schools to emphasize prevention of illness and healthy lifestyles. These policies would help to prevent the ever-rising costs of health care that currently burden the budgets of cities and states.

What is a telomere and its role in the limits of human life span?

A telomere is the short ending of a chromosome. It has been compared to the ends of a shoelace as an analogy. The telomere has been found to be longer in people with longer life spans and shorter in those with limited life span. The telomere length may be influenced by nutritional factors, stress, and other behaviors. Certain diets will cause the telomeres to become shorter over time. A diet that is rich in refined sugar, sucrose, fructose, and syrups is one. Inflammatory diets, or diets that increase oxidative stress and include red meats, processed meats, white bread, sodas, saturated fats, omega-6 polyunsaturated fats, heavy alcohol consumption, and excessive iron supplements also shorten telomeres. These diets may be shortening your life and health span as well.

To know more about the telomeres, I want you to review chapter 2, particularly the section on telomeres. Today you can find many companies offering testing of telomeres. This information may be used as guidance to modify your lifestyle and increase the levels of telomerase, the enzyme that helps to increase the length of the telomeres. Check Appendix G, "Resources," for names of such companies.

The good news is that we can do something to experience good health and have a healthier life span beyond those years. All is within our reach if we can lengthen our telomeres by a proper diet and behaviors. Preventing premature chronological aging and moving into a younger biological cellular age is possible and within reach. This is what matters—moving from the fast lane of chronological age into the slower and healthier lane of biological cellular age. These extraordinary findings explain why reversing aging is possible. As suggested previously, in the near future, we may be able to find centenarians who look twenty or thirty years or more years younger than their actual chronological age.

This is the basis of this book. My prescription is a guide to maintain a healthy biological cellular system without drugs to expand life span to limits that we have not seen yet. It may be possible, if we start early, to expand the limits of the Hayflick effect by encouraging our telomeres to remain longer and, thus, enabling our cells to live longer and to divide a few more cycles. It may be possible to increase the telomerase levels by a combination of nutrients and genetic interventions to prolong the life span of all cells. Another key factor is the expansion and vitality of the immune system. People may die young with a weakened immune system even though the cells are young and healthy. We should be reminded that children die of infectious diseases when the immune system fails to protect them. Strengthening the stem cells and the immune system is an important component of a healthy lifestyle. Stress has been recognized as a stressor that may lower our capacity to fight infection and our life span. Through bioresilience, we may be able to expand our existence in case we are confronted with any infection threatening our existence at any point in our life spans. This is why a strong immune system and a healthier biological cellular system is what matters.

Recent research that shows the damage done by sugar confirms our suspicion that refined sugar, syrups, and many other foods that damage our DNA and telomeres—or decrease the levels of telomerase—in our chromosomes are the enemies. These toxic foods continue to do so much damage not only to us but also to humanity. This epiphany and the good health and younger look of my wife are some of the factors that motivated me to write this book. My wife and I feel that, if we can help other people by sharing our good ideas and life experiences and my many years of practicing medicine, we have accomplished something that may live as a legacy for future generations. Eventually, we hope we can create a movement to protect future generations and stop the damage done by the consumption of refined sugars, harmful carbohydrates, bad fats, and unhealthy foods, which are the cause of genetic mutations, premature aging, and disease.

Can we live longer and reverse aging?

Yes, definitely, we can. Research is advancing at a fast pace to meet this objective. *Living Longer and Reversing Aging* offers a prescription or a pathway to reach the destination of a lifestyle of wellness. You can start at anytime to experience the benefits of this healthier lifestyle by following the steps outlined in my prescription. This is lifestyle medicine, which I hope may become a specialty, one day.

If you want to be more inquisitive and have the money to invest in your health, I recommend having a physical, including a complete nutritional and hormonal assessment to know more about your deficiencies or imbalances. Bringing your body to a perfect balance will restore the feedback mechanism in your hormonal system, normalize you circadian rhythms, improve and strengthen your immune system, restore the normal production of hormones to repair the damage already done by any deficiency, and reverse the ongoing aging process.

The most exciting biological treatments available to reverse aging are blood products and stem cells. Blood or plasma from young individuals or umbilical cords provides mesenchymal stem cells that help the body rejuvenate itself. These are expensive therapies available in many countries except the United States, where there are restrictions from the FDA. Before considering these therapies, people interested in this form of rejuvenation should consider other therapies to rejuvenate old stem cells. A few avenues to try include:

1. mTOR inhibition with rapamycin
2. boosting cellular AMPK activity
3. increasing NAD+ levels
4. activating sirtuin proteins

NAD+ activity can be improved by taking nicotinamide riboside, a precursor of NAD+ as a supplement, 250 to 750 mg a day.

AMPK can be increased by caloric restriction and reducing sugars in particular. AMPK activators are available as supplements in the market. Metformin, curcumin (turmeric), green tea, matcha, and aerobic exercise are helpful to increase AMPK.

To increase SIRT1 expression, you can use resveratrol, 100 to 250 mg a day.

The combined benefit of all these supplements, exercise, and reduced caloric intake is favorable to promote stem cell health, from improving self-renewal to regenerative capacity. All these supplements are available in health food stores. Keeping your current and old stem cells healthy is a way to reverse aging and maintain a strong immune system.

The Long Life Family Study sponsored by the National Institutes of Health is investigating which genetic, environmental, and behavioral factors contribute to longevity. In the most recent census, health officials predicted that, by 2050, more that one million people will be over a hundred years old. It is expected that the majority of these centenarians will be mentally alert, full of vigor and energy, free of disability, and eager to enjoy a life to the fullest. Researchers are studying the traditional lifestyle and behaviors that contribute to a healthier longevity. The New England Centenary Study, of 850 centenarians, has identified some traits that contribute to longevity. They include no smoking, being extroverted, and having a lean body.

Geneticists and biologists have been investigating the secrets of longevity at the cellular level. Their goal is to identify the genes associated with aging and chronic illness. Advances in genomic technology now allow doctors to connect specific genes to bodily functions. These findings will lead to the discovery of compounds, nutrients, peptides, and medicines that can modify the genes to delay aging or stop a degenerative illness. Dr. David Sinclair from Harvard Medical School said, "We are going through a revolution." He cofounded Sitris, a biotech company developing antiaging compounds to improve health. It is expected that we will see many companies, researchers, and scientists involved in this type of research to extend longevity. One of these companies is Juvenescence created by Jim Mellon and Al Chalabi. Juvenescence is investing in new technologists and research to extend human life span and reverse aging. Mellon and Chalabi have a vision of a better life ahead and the benefits of research into longevity science.

The framework to build the bridge to take you to this new world of longevity and wellness is explained in *Living Longer and Reversing Aging*. You don't have to wait several decades for new research. You can start now, since my recommendations are easy to follow and provide the structure for a healthier lifestyle. Millions are already looking for ways to change their lifestyles so they can live longer and reverse aging. In the future, there will be lifestyle wellness communities where all members will meet and become selective in the foods they eat, share ideas similar to the ones described in my DRESS-SS prescription, and come together to improve their health and attain longer life spans. You should stay informed and join these groups to learn more about how to improve your health and enjoy a life of wellness and happiness. If some new developments, nutrients, supplements, medical compounds, or technologies come along to increase your longevity, you will already be ahead.

Research continues, and until more safe and definite compounds or agents are available, the steps outlined in my DRESS-SS prescription are your best guides to follow at this time.

Several pharmaceutical agents, such as Metformin to treat diabetes, have been tested to extend life span and delay aging-related diseases. If you are already diabetic, taking Metformin may lessen other diseases and may help to prolong your life span. If you are not diabetic, I don't recommend using this drug at this time. Decreasing insulin resistance through a good diet, weight control, caloric restriction, pharmaceuticals, minerals like chromium and zinc, cinnamon, berberine, alpha lipoid acid, AMPK activators, and a healthy gut microbiome are better alternatives. One of the good bacteria to improve metabolic health is *Akkermansia muciniphila*. This bacteria has shown beneficial actions to improve diabetes and prevent obesity. Metformin boosts the amount of this bacteria in the gut according to recent research. Check your probiotics to select good bacteria for a healthy gut.

Since telomeres shorten with an improper diet or stress, it is important to pay attention to any nutritional deficiencies and internal stressors responsible for their shortening and a shorter life span.

You need to see a qualified doctor to request lab work to determine what types of deficiencies you have. Your doctor can guide you in use the best kind of supplements, hormones, or pharmaceutical agents you need to reach your ultimate goal of optimal health. Checking the length of your telomeres is also important to assess your progress and your diet program. Fortunately, today many labs provide this service at reasonable cost. (See the resources section at the end of the book.) A baseline test to determine your telomere's length is important. Follow-up testing every two or three years may be necessary to assess your progress. Unfortunately, many doctors have no interest in helping patients to know more about their telomeres' health or nutritional deficiencies. I recommend searching for doctors with additional training in complementary and alternative Medicine, if your family doctor or internist is unwilling to help you. In Appendix G, I provide a list of laboratories that perform these tests.

You also may need lab testing to check your white and red cells to be sure you do not have anemia secondary to an iron or vitamin deficiency. Additional testing to check your liver, kidneys, electrolytes, minerals, and vitamin levels may help to evaluate you overall health. Men should have a PSA testing to check the prostate for the possibility of cancer. To cut the cost of testing, my clinic and many other labs offer online testing at affordable prices. Check the resources section for more information. Women should continue to have Pap smears and mammograms to prevent cancer from developing. It takes time to reverse changes related to aging and the signs and symptoms associated with them. If you continue to be alarmed at the symptoms you're experiencing, you should visit your doctor so he or she can determine and diagnose if you have a thyroid, estrogen, testosterone, iron, or other hormone or mineral deficiency.

As I said before, not all doctors are aware of these changes, and some are reluctant to address nutritional deficiencies to help you bring your body into a perfect equilibrium. They instead give their patients Valium, sleeping pills, and antidepressants, when the real problems are metabolic changes due to internal deficiencies; insulin resistance; poor diets; allergies to milk or milk products, gluten, or pollens and dust; and low hormone levels that lead to age-related diseases and premature aging.

A few words of warning: Doctors usually rely on laboratory values provided by labs with a wide range of variability. A low normal thyroid value may be insufficient for someone who is having symptoms of hypothyroidism. The doctor may not check whether there is a deficiency of iron or iodine that may be contributing to a low thyroid as we described before. An incomplete or limited test may miss valuable information about your problem or deficiency. The same is true for men with erectile dysfunction (ED). The normal lab report of 300 mg/ml of total testosterone in a man with symptoms of low T at age fifty is misleading, and the man can go undertreated and remain unable to have normal erections, when the normal range of testosterone for him may be twice the level reported by the lab. The mistake, made by many doctors, is to treat the lab result and not the patient.

The same is true for women entering menopause. Many doctors are unwilling to provide hormone replacement therapy to a woman. There is a place to provide bio-identical hormones for the symptoms of menopause, as long as there is no history of cancer or genetic predisposition to cancer of the ovaries and breasts, or a positive BRCA1 and BRCA2 genetic test.

Giving a man with low T injectable testosterone for two weeks to raise his levels will determine if the ED can go away. If a man is experiencing normal erections with the increased levels of testosterone, the clinical response is the best way to assess the treatment.

The same principle applies to diet and the use of mineral and supplements. We may need additional supplements to help our cells and organs stay in optimal shape at different times of our life cycles. My approach to staying healthy, delaying premature aging, and increasing longevity is to assess and reevaluate every six to twelve months for changes to correct deficiencies and to become aware of internal changes or diseases that can affect your health. The office visit is also an opportunity to learn through education, healthy practices, and actions to reach optimal health and happiness.

Can we expect a better future?

The journey to stop cancer, arthritis, heart disease, and many other illnesses continues every day. Very soon, we will be able to conquer many of the problems that shorten our life and health span. New treatments and new drugs are in the process of development to conquer many chronic illnesses and cancer. The future is promising, and we expect life spans to increase, as was the case with the antibiotic revolution. We have to prepare to live longer—beyond a hundred years of age. My DRESS-SS prescription is my best advice to you and your family on how to reach an old age in the best possible form mentally and physically. My prescription is the beginning of a better life and a healthy longevity. You should view life like a marathon, where you are expected to reach the goal line in the best possible shape. I want you to think that way. I am sure you want to age gracefully and enjoy life, walking unassisted and breathing on your own without the aid of an oxygen tank when you reach the goal line. I believe most of us want to reach old age healthier and looking many years younger than our peers of the same chronological age. There is no reason you cannot achieve these goals.

You need to develop awareness of these steps and follow my prescription to guide you so that you can make good choices. You should believe in yourself and make this possible. You also need to educate yourself about what is best for you to stay healthy and take action. Thinking but failing to act is not an option. Procrastinating is not a solution. You need discipline and determination to make this change possible. Your life and a happier, healthy longevity are in your hands. My book is a guide to help you reach your ultimate goal for optimal health. It does not matter how old you are; it's time to begin to assess your health, make changes, and act. I encourage you to start today. Keep this book with you all the time. Get the digital version to check anything you want when you have a break, when buying groceries, or when traveling. This book has a great deal of information that can make you happier and help you live longer. Share this information with your friends and family. If you are a couple, make this book an essential guide to maintain a healthier lifestyle. Remember, happiness is the ultimate goal. I want you to use this book to enhance your health and level of happiness. If you can add a few more years to your life and live healthier, delay aging, and be happier, you should feel rewarded. The younger you start to assess your health and habits, determine what changes you should make, and live a healthier lifestyle, the greater the reward.

As we age, we also grow in wisdom, and this wisdom will become a gift to humankind and the younger generations. As we age, we mature and grow spiritually, as well. This mature spirituality is a blessing for you, your loved ones, your friends, and humanity. I have no doubt that boomers who are living longer will have a significant influence on how we will live in the future. As millions of people pay more attention to their health, more knowledge and changes for the better will come their way. Currently, boomers contribute more than $7 trillion to the economy. In fifteen more years, the impact of their contributions will surpass $20 trillion. Prolonging age and years of gainful activity and wisdom may become a bonanza for families; companies; the national economy; teaching institutions engaged in research, science, and medicine; and better health care for many nations.

Start this longevity revolution today. Begin by being aware of how to improve your health and how to correct deficiencies. Remember that, by keeping your body healthy through positive actions, you will also improve your mind and spirit. Keeping your body healthy at the cellular level is an important concept that will help keep your organ functions in check for a perfect balance; through this balance, you will achieve good health, stay younger, and live longer. Elite athletes, Olympic men and women, should use this book and my prescription to achieve strength, optimal health, and endurance in order to be successful in any competitive sport. The more your mind and body are in perfect equilibrium, the greater your success.

DRESS-SS is my prescription for living a healthy, long life and reversing aging. I also call this prescription a code or formula for a better life or a healthier lifestyle. This is your foundation for healthy and joyful living. Although diet is very important, diet alone is not enough. You need to build on this foundation by introducing rest, exercise, healthy sleep, and stress management into your daily routine. This is the basic structure for a healthy, happy, satisfied lifestyle.

CONCLUSION

Bringing it all together

The path to living longer and reversing aging is a lifestyle of wellness that maintains a healthy brain and body. A healthy brain ensures a healthy mind and body. A balanced brain will allow you to remain smart and attentive, be able to remember short- and long-term memories, and remain calm and happy throughout your life span. All this requires a positive attitude and a desire to change your lifestyle. This book provides the prescription and steps to make meaningful changes to your lifestyle if you want to reach an old age looking younger and healthier. Remember that biological age is more important than chronological age for optimal cognitive and physical health.

For my prescription for healthier living, I investigated many sources to make this book possible. When I decided to undertake this project, I felt the need to research books, articles, magazines, websites, and the internet for more information about brain power, diets, and longevity. I was happily surprised about the universal interest in living healthier and longer.

Ongoing research to understand the development of atherosclerosis and heart attacks by foods in our diets is important to prevent the number one cause of death in men and women in the United States. What I found interesting is the fact that diets rich in carbohydrates and, particularly, refined sugar appear to have some relationship with the development of cancer. As a doctor, I never thought sugar might be related to cancer. As a professor of medicine, I never heard any of my colleagues talk about this relationship or the damage done to our mitochondria or DNA by free radicals. A great deal of research is going on in this area, and it is promising. I personally believe we are not far away from linking our dietary habits with cancer and many genetic diseases.

What is also interesting is the use of nutrients and diets to modify our genome or gene defects. The experiments done in 2000 at Duke University with yellow fur mice that carry the agouti gene are very revealing. Dr. Michael Murray, in *The Magic of Food*, reports how good nutrition lowers the risk of genetic disease expression (Murray 2017, 3). In a 2000 landmark study at Duke University, researchers found that fat mice with yellow fur carry the agouti gene, which made them fat and yellow. This gene increases dramatically their risk to develop cancer and diabetes. Before mice were conceived, a test group of mother mice was fed a diet rich in Vitamin B12, folic acid, and SAM-e. The baby mice were born brown and slender and as they matured didn't succumb to cancer and diabetes. The nutritional intervention in the mother's diet had completely erased the cancerous, diabetic genetic destiny of the agouti mice. Although the brown mice had the same genome as the yellow mice, the expression of the genome was significantly different because of nutritional factors.

This is another instance of the magic of food and proof that genetic tendencies can be changed with dietary and nutritional approaches. We already know that deficiencies of folic acid in the pregnant mother may lead to brain and nerve defects for the child. There are many other diseases or problems in which a nutritional deficiency leads to a genetic defect or the expression of a defective gene. In chapter 2, "D is for Diet," I mentioned the healing powers of some diets. Ketogenic diets have a definite benefit for children with epilepsy or seizure disorders. They may also explain why people on these diets can reverse type 2 diabetes or prevent some neurological illnesses. Unfortunately as you age, the body begins to change before you realize that the brain speed and function begins to change as well. If you ignore the body changes as determined by hormonal changes, your brain will begin to experience greater decline. The gradual progressive cognitive decline associated with an aging brain and body exists in a continuum. The good news is that, with proper assessment of our diets, nutrients, and hormonal levels, we can bring our bodies and minds to an optimal balance for improved function. A healthier mind leads to greater joy and a life of greater love and happiness.

A longevity revolution is at hand, and I expect to see an expansion of the limits of human life span in the next fifty years. Our life span is now limited to 120 years, probably due to many factors related to diets and the many stresses of modern life. My prescription is a guide to modify the current limits and to provide a better pathway or a bridge to a healthier existence and longevity. We continue to learn more about our genes every day. The human genome has been unraveled, and every day we know more about our genes and their functions. Understanding cellular function and the genes is the way to improve our health and life spans. We are learning from other mammals who live longer what genes or factors allow them to live hundreds of years more than us, as is the case with the turtles, fish, and reptiles. Why can animals like the Mexican salamander regenerate limbs or organs?

Eventually, we will be able to develop a map of the genes responsible for aging. Very likely, many of these genes can be modified and become rejuvenated with adjustment of nutrients in our diets before the genes begin to fail. Some other genes may be modified with drugs or specific interventions. Some of these drugs already under research are available and in use. The most promising, so far are metformin and rapamycin. These drugs and many other compounds eventually will help to prolong or delay aging. Without question, our bodies at the cellular level have been under a great deal of stress by oxidative damage from harmful diets that produce thousands of damaging free radicals. The consumption of excessive sugars from early age have been damaging our DNA and mitochondria, causing alterations in the gene sequences leading to mutations resulting in cancers and degenerative diseases. The way to fight these constant attacks is for us to remain vigilant and eat foods that can prevent and help to repair the damage. Eating foods rich in antioxidants is one way to control the damage. Reducing caloric intake as we age has been found to prolong life spans. Rebalancing our hormones as we age is another way to keep our systems functioning as normally as possible. Adding selective micronutrients, minerals, to prevent deficits of metabolic functions may help to prevent further damage. The goal is to maintain a healthy cellular system that is working at top shape all the time. The benefit is good health; less inflammation; which is damaging; and less or no DNA and mitochondrial damage.

As we advance in survival in our planet, we may have to consider how to live longer if we decide to explore other planets. Space exploration and travel is now possible. To survive the rigors of space travel and ensure our survival on other planets, we must continue to find ways to extend our life spans and improve our health here, on our own planet, first. Research will continue to accelerate, and we will find ways to expand and improve our health by learning more about our genome and genetic sequencing to bring and maintain balance at the cellular level before a deficiency or mutation develops.

Today we enjoy ways to assess our bodies and find proper diets, supplements, and vitamins to compensate for any deficiencies, and my DRESS-SS prescription is your pathway to live longer and healthier every day of your life, in this new world of wellness and longer life spans.

I hope that *Living Longer and Reversing Aging* brings more attention to the role of nutrients and diets in our genes and overall cellular functions and their effect on our health by my colleagues in medicine. As clinicians, we must learn more about the effects of nutritional imbalances that may lead to illness. As I indicated previously chapters 1 and 2, physicians many times don't realize the effects a medication is causing in relation to the absorption of many nutrients. Diuretics may cause a depletion of magnesium and vitamins necessary for many metabolic processes. Normal lab results may not mean that the patient is healthy. A subtle deficiency may be sufficient for a person to feel tired or weak. The same is true for patients undergoing surgery. A person should be in a positive nutritional balance before surgery to prevent complications, infections, and delayed healing. My early experience with parenteral nutrition was very useful to see the benefits of a proper balanced nutrition. Understanding the genes involved in aging will play a big role in treating many degenerative diseases, heart disease, and cancer and in the prevention of a weakened immune system.

During my research of the literature, I found different studies that evaluated cholesterol and fats in the development of heart disease. Many renowned scientists and physicians have conducted long-term studies, sometimes with different results. It is difficult for a practicing physician to ascertain who is correct when one study contradicts the other or when a reputed organization recommends a diet, only to find out it was the wrong recommendation years later.

The quest to decrease the formation of plaque in arteriosclerosis continues. Among the recommendations by Dr. Ornish and Dr. Esselstyn, Pritikin, Dr. Fuhrman, Dr. Guntry, and more recently Dr. Valter Longo's longevity diet, I found something in common. This is, the importance of using less bad fats in our diets to prevent the formation of plaque and a means to reverse this process. The problem I found is that some of these diets are too rigid and difficult to follow. Another problem is the confusion about fat intake. As more recent research demonstrates, not all foods or fats are bad. In fact, Dr. Longo feels that olive oil, fish, nuts, and other plant-based foods are good, something Dr. Esselstyn doesn't allow (Esselstyn 2008). Clinicians, like me, would appreciate more clarity and more research to make recommendations more practical.

I personally believe that Dr. Longo's longevity diet is closer to what a clinician can recommend (Longo 2018). His diet is basically a modified Mediterranean diet, or plant-based diet, low in pasta, bread, and fruits. A plant-based diet is the benchmark. According to many of these researchers, their diets don't include much meat, given the fact that many researchers have deemed meat the culprit of many problems. This was confirmed by a Harvard study of men and women on low-carbohydrate diets rich in animal fat, where participants had a 40 percent higher risk of dying of cardiovascular disease than those on low-fat diets. I recommend meat only once a month or not at all. Fish consumption is still good, since it provides omega-3, an essential fatty acid for cell function.

In *The Plant Paradox*, Steven Guntry, MD, considers lectins in legumes, whole grains, and meat products the source of many health problems and, in particular, coronary artery disease. This issue was extensively described in the chapter for diet.

Lots of scientific research now points to a diet low in animal fats to extend life, which is more favorable to a healthy longevity. We have to become selective with all the fats we consume. Lectin-containing fats prevalent in the American diet and the oils from soy, cottonseed, sunflower, canola, corn, grape seed, and peanut, all contain high levels of polyunsaturated omega-6 fats, which trigger an inflammatory cascade in the coronary arteries. Diets rich in lectins and WGA present in whole grains cause CAD.

Good fats are not dangerous, as was believed years ago. They include olive oil, coconut oil, MCT oil, perilla oil, avocado oil, sesame oil, cod liver oil, and macadamia oil. There has been a great deal of misinformation from reputable organizations, which has done harm to millions of people and created lots of confusion.

I don't find anything wrong with vitamin and mineral supplementation on a daily basis, even though some national organizations disagree and don't recommend adding vitamins and supplements to a diet. It is well documented that women need additional iron, folic acid, and minerals during pregnancy and breastfeeding. As we age, there must be a need of constant reassessment of our lipids, micronutrients, and hormones, since their levels change as function of different organs decline. As we age, certain medications deplete the body of many nutrients and minerals, which in turn causes symptoms many doctors ignore because they are not interested in nutrition or the side effects of these medications. I personally believe children, women, athletes, seniors, and people taking medications require supplementation to prevent nutritional deficiencies and symptoms.

This is the case with cholesterol-lowering drugs, which cause deficiencies of CoQ10 in the mitochondria, resulting in symptoms like muscle cramps, body aches, and joint pain. This is something many physicians ignore. Rather than prescribing opioids, the solution is to decrease the dose of the drug and prescribe CoQ10 as a supplement to relieve pain. The same is true for many other drugs that may cause all kinds of pain and inflammation. The tendency to prescribe opioids has to be reassessed by the medical profession. The easy solution—providing the narcotic without assessing the long-term consequences—is not acceptable. There are supplements like turmeric, SAM-e, and CoQ10 and others that help to relieve pain without dependency. More genetic research is necessary to help people with chronic pain and to eliminate the need of narcotic analgesics. Precision and lifestyle medicine is the way to solve this problem.

Insurance companies and government entities should allow insurance companies to pay for genetic testing to find the correct medicine and the use of supplements to keep people healthy, rather than on narcotics, which may lead to dependency and death. The same is true for a balanced education in schools and nutritional counseling to start the elimination of many sugars in processed foods. There should be a law prohibiting giving sugary drinks or juices to children below age two. Any sugary drink sold should not have more than 15 g of sugar. Syrups should be limited to no more than 10 g of carbohydrates. Warnings about the dangers of syrups containing fructose and excessive sugars must be part of the labeling. Fines to manufacturers violating these limits should be in place. Taxing any product exceeding an acceptable minimum of sugars could be a solution, helping to decrease the addiction to sugar and long-term health consequences and costs associated with the care of those affected by the excessive consumption of sugars.

Making people responsible for their health is also important. The cost of caring for people with obesity, metabolic syndrome, and heart disease is staggering. Promoting a healthy lifestyle saves money at the family and national level.

We are at the threshold of a longevity revolution and should pay more attention to wellness and healthy lifestyles. It is not impossible for a human being to look decades younger than his or her chronological age or to live to be 150. As more discoveries are made to cure cancer, heart disease, diabetes, and chronic illnesses, it is very possible to live beyond 100. The key is to reach this age in the best possible health, with all mental faculties and body in great shape. Dying healthy beyond 100 may become an acceptable reality and a goal that is not possible today. I believe that lifestyle medicine, with emphasis in wellness and healthier cell biology, may become an important specialty, where people could find the best doctors who can guide them to reach a life of wellness and longer, healthier life spans.

I have placed emphasis on diet as my first letter of DRESS-SS because we are what we eat to a great extent. As we learn how micronutrients affect cell functions, we will be able to select better foods, which will help us to reverse aging and many genetic defects. A good diet should help to keep our immune system strong and ready to fight infections and cancers.

But diet alone is not the solution. Our bodies are complex and require sufficient exercise to prevent deterioration of our organs. Exercise increases blood flow to tissues, providing more oxygen and nutrients to all the cells. Increased blood flow allows the removal of toxic materials resulting from metabolic cellular processes. Exercise also provides a feeling of well-being and helps to burn excessive calories consumed. Our brains benefit from daily exercise to maintain important neurological functions, memory, and intellectual activity. After a stroke and the loss of brain cells, the brain stem cells may repair damaged connections to improve muscle function, balance, and coordination. Exercise is a great way to fight obesity and improve heart function after a heart attack. Many centers offer cardiac rehabilitation programs to help those with loss of cardiac function after a heart attack.

As human beings, we are subject to emotions and feelings, which affect our overall health. Resting and sleeping give our bodies time to repair damage and prepare the body for further action. Controlling stress is very important to prevent damage to our health. As a physician, I believe a majority of complaints in a doctor's office are related to stress. In my book, I offer recommendations to manage stress.

In closing, I can't dismiss the beneficial effects of spirituality. If you are not a believer, you are missing an important component of the wholeness of the individual. Fighting or stressing to deny and accept this component of our being is foolish. There is more to gain than to lose when we accept the value of spirituality. Human beings are very special, and for some reason, we have evolved to the top of the biological world.

As a doctor, I wish those using my prescription a life of better health, throughout their life spans. If you follow this prescription, you can expect a life of wellness that will allow you to live longer and look younger. We are at the threshold of a longevity revolution, and this book is your guide and the bridge to getting there in better shape, full of joy and gratitude.

Living Longer and Reversing Aging is the key to finding the elusive fountain of health and youth. Keep this book at hand; it is my legacy to help people to stay healthy and well. A wellness approach to health is better than the traditional sickness model. Empowering the individual to take care of himself or herself will provide beneficial results to the individual, physically, emotionally, and financially. A new world of lifestyle wellness and longer longevity is waiting for you. Millions are moving toward this world of wellness every day. They are exercising, eating healthy, and taking vitamins and supplements to stay healthy and live longer. This book is a source of information to guide anyone who wants to improve his or her health and reach a longer life span. Research is advancing at a very fast pace. Scientists are working to improve our lives on this planet, and investors are using their money to accelerate the pace of this research and expansion of this new world of lifestyle wellness. Stem cell research is helping to repair damaged tissues and organs. Medicines like metformin appear to protect against heart disease, cancer, possibly Alzheimer's, and other diseases of aging. Many more compounds are in the process of development as well. A permanent state of wellness lowers the cost of medical care at the family and state level. Along the way, remember to find love and happiness to make your existence on this planet the most joyful experience of all time.

ILLUSTRATIONS

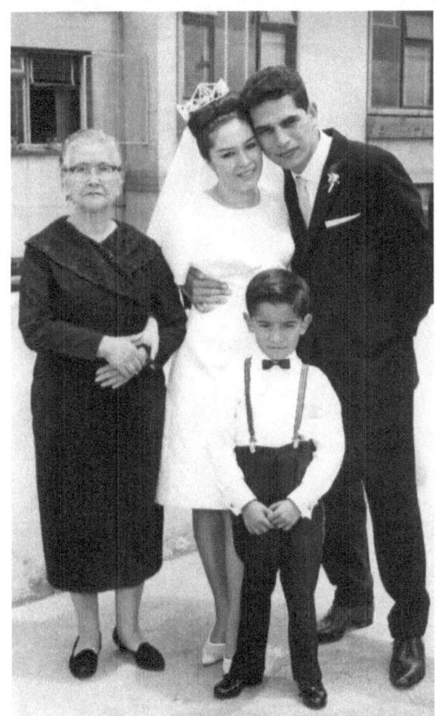

Clara's Grandmother age 73, Clara, Jairo and
William, Jairo's younger brother. July 1965

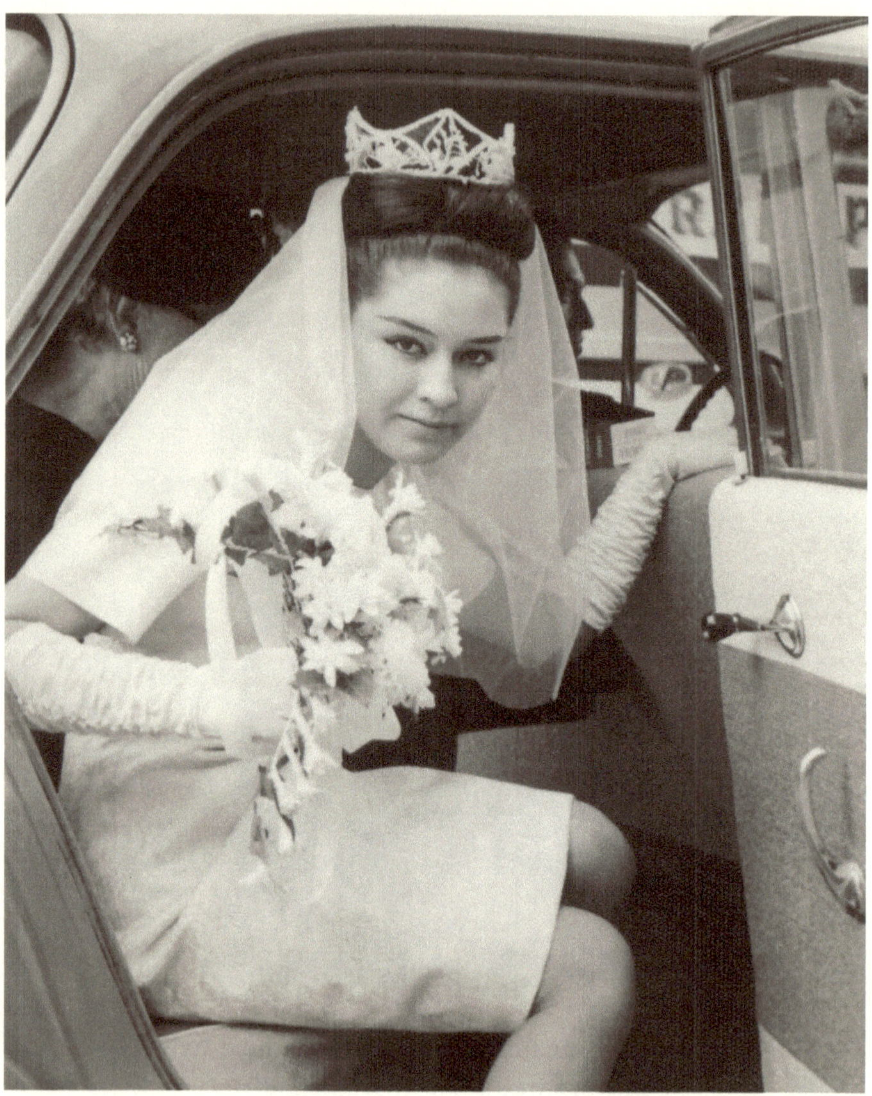

Picture 2. Jairo and Clara's wedding

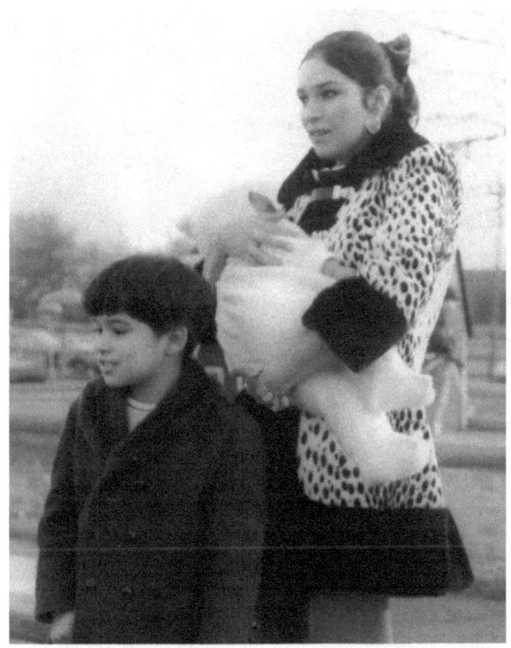

Picture 3. Clara and children 1970

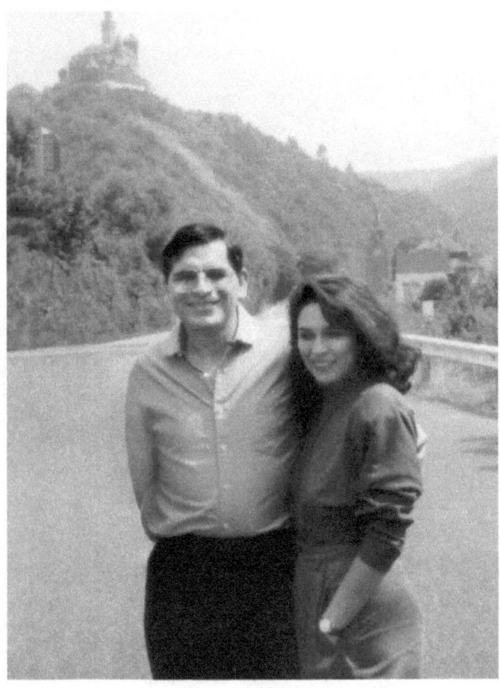

Picture 4. Jairo and Clara in the '80s

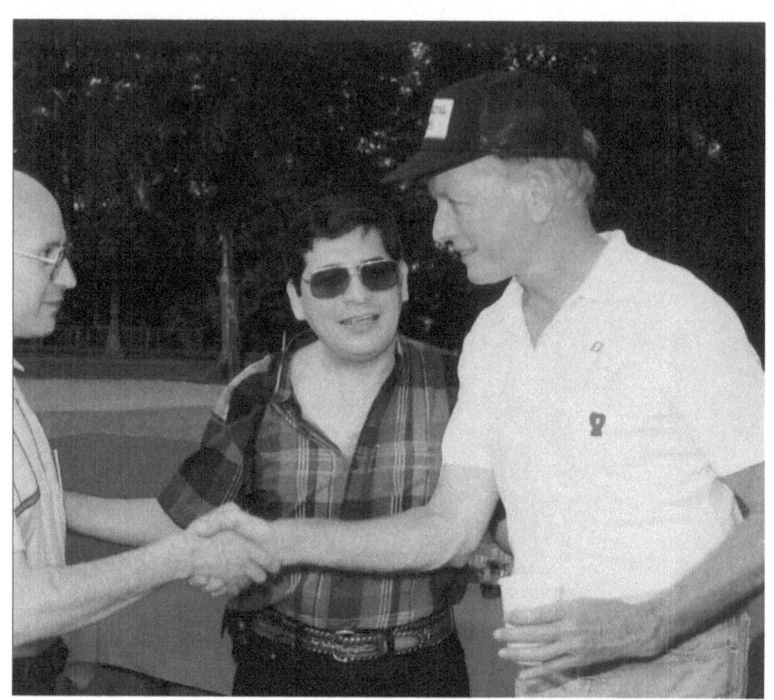

Picture 5. Jairo and Dr Denton Cooley

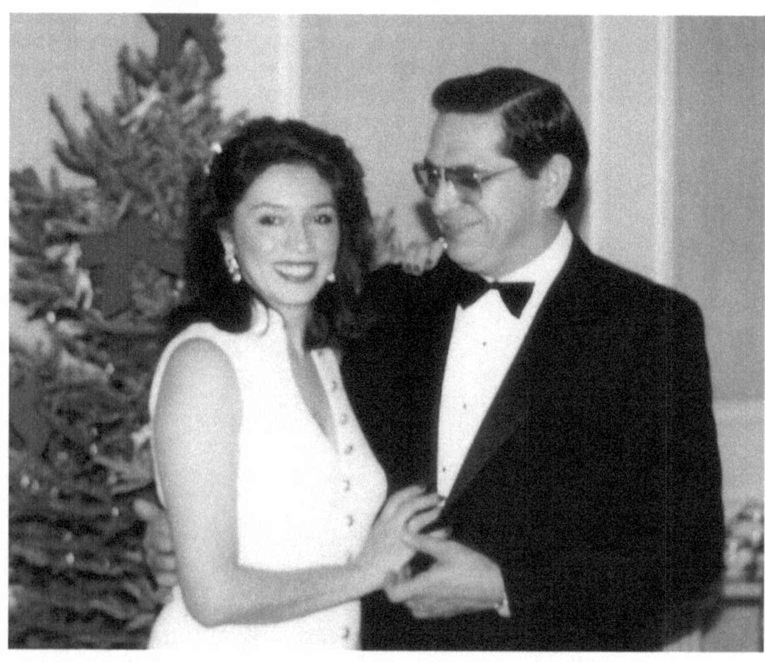

Picture 6. Jairo and Clara, 1990.

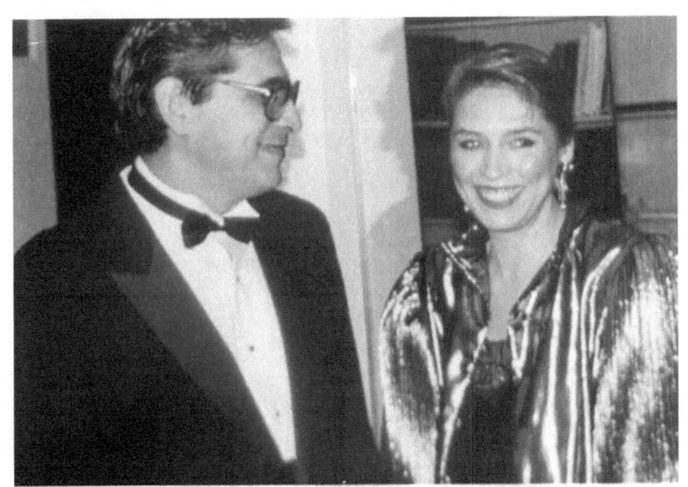

Picture 7. Jairo and Clara, 2000

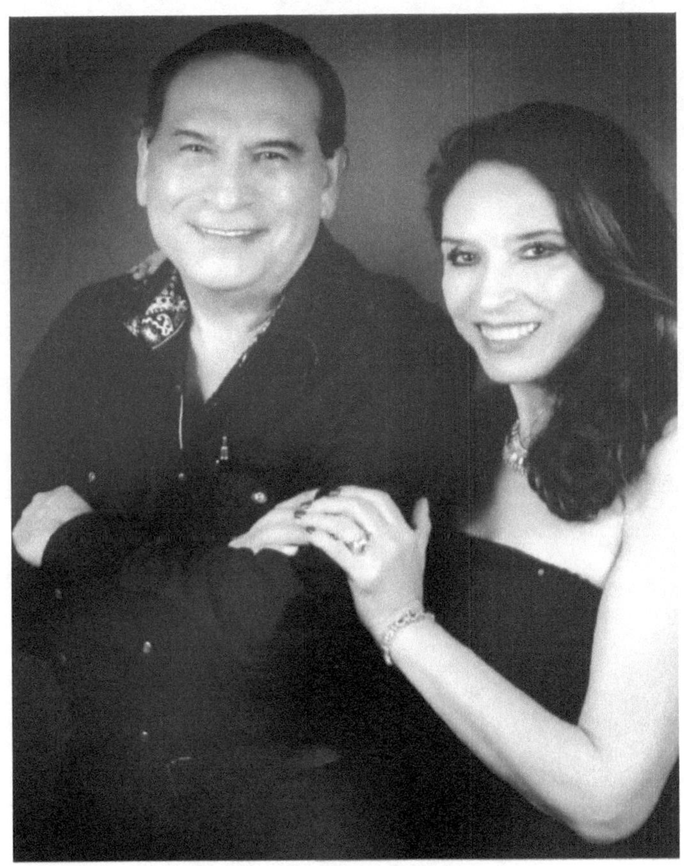

Picture 8. Jairo and Clara, 2015

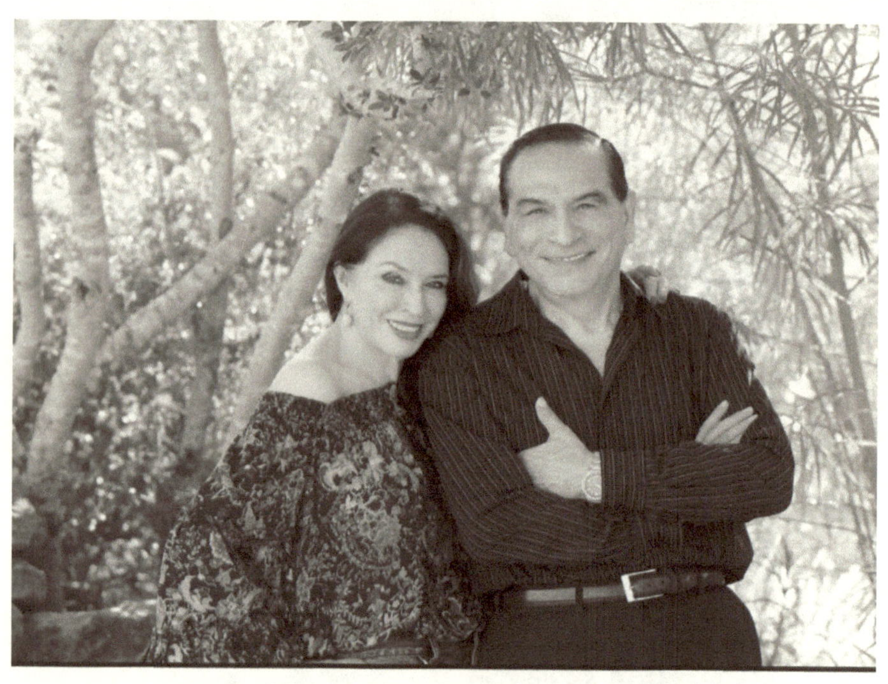

Picture 9. Jairo and Clara, 2018

APPENDIX A

Supplements for Better Health

This list details supplements I usually recommend in my practice. I selected products that my patients report to be beneficial. I do not endorse any brands. However, I have listed some brands that I feel have been very effective. Before taking supplements, you should check with your doctor for any interaction with other medicines you take. Many supplements may affect clotting and bleeding time, so you should check with your doctor before surgery. It is better to discontinue your supplements before surgery to prevent complications. You may resume them as soon as is safe after surgery.

This is a partial list of supplements I recommend. There are many products and combinations that are also effective. I usually recommend a combination for better results. I use a code of stars to indicate which products and combinations are more effective and earn my highest recommendation. One star (*) has the lowest rating, and four stars (****) is the highest recommendation.

All these products are available in health food stores.

Joint Health, Pain Relief, and Inflammation Supplements

- Curcumin by CuraMed – BCM 95 soft gels; twice a day ****
- Turmeric Supreme by Gaia Herbs – Contains black pepper for better absorption; one cap twice a day ****
- Turmeric powder – Sprinkle in salads, cereals, or any other foods; good supplement for the joints, brain function, and pain **

- SAM-e 400 mg by Jarrow Formulas – One tab twice a day; helps to support connective tissue and brain function and is good for pain relief****
- CoQ10 – One 200 mg cap a day; good supplement if you are taking statins to lower cholesterol***
- Q-absorb (CoQ10) by Jarrow Formulas – 100 mg; one or two caps a day; helps to prevent and reduce joint and muscle pain associated with the intake of cholesterol-lowering medicines ****
- Glucosamine Chondroitin MSM caps – One a day; helps build cartilage, particularly of knees ****
- Ultimate Omega – 1,280 mg of omega-3 soft gels; one a day ****
- Omega-3 from fish oil – Comes in liquid with excellent flavors. Barlean brand (mango, passion fruit, and orange); one teaspoon in a half glass of orange juice provides two essential nutrients (omega-3, an essential fatty acid, and vitamin C) ****
- Vitamin D3 – 2,000 IU; one soft gel a day ****

Other Helpful Supplements for the Joints and Pain

- Alpha Lipoic Acid 600 mg by Doctor's Best – one cap a day ****
- Omega-3 Krill Oil 1000 mg by Megared – one cap a day ****
- Hydraplenish by Nature's Way – hyaluronic acid; one cap a day ***
- ZYFLAMEND Whole Body by New Chapter – one capsule a day; contains several herbs to relieve inflammation and pain ***

For Headaches

- Feverfew – one cap twice a day**
- Migelief by Quantum Health – one tab twice a day**

Migraines

- Magnesium – 400 mg caps; one a day ***
- CoQ10 – 200 mg; once a day ***
- Vitamin B complex – one cap a day ***

Supplements to lower insulin resistance and improve diabetes

- Cinnamon extract 1,000 mg tabs by Natrol – one tab a day***
- Alpha Lipoic Acid 600 mg by Doctor's Best – one cap a day****
- Zinc – 30 mg tab, once a day ***
- Chromium picolinate – 500 mcg a day****
- AMPK tablets from Life Extension – one tablet a day****
- Berberine tablets from Solaray – 500 mg a day****

Supplements to raise HDL and lower triglycerides

- Yeast flakes by Kalvitamins ****
- Chromium picolinate 500 mcg a day ****

Supplements for stress and energy

- Ashwagandha caps by Himalaya – one cap twice a day ****
- Gotu kola by Now – one cap a day ****
- GABA chewable tablets – one tab twice a day ***
- Triple-Tea Fat Burner by Irwin – one cap in the morning ***
- Adrenal health by Gaia Herbs – Contains holy basil and *Rhodiola*; two caps twice a day ***
- Echinacea *angustifolia* root extract tablets ****

Osteoporosis and arthritis prevention

- Sunlight fifteen minutes a day
- A diet rich in salmon, oysters, fish, sardines, low-fat milk, cheese, and green vegetables
- Calcium supplements
- Vitamin D3 – 2,000 units twice a day ****
- Calcium, magnesium, vitamin D liquid – one teaspoon a day ****
- Adequate intake of minerals, such as magnesium, calcium, potassium, zinc, and vitamin K

Sleep supplements

Take one or use a combination of these as needed:

- Magnesium 400 mg – one capsule at bedtime ****
- Tart cherry – one capsule at night ***
- Power to Sleep Capsules – one an hour before bedtime***
- Melatonin 3 mg Fast Action – one tablet one hour before bedtime ****
- Valerian tea – 1 to 2 brewed bags at bedtime ***
- Nightly Night Tea – 1 to 2 brewed bags at bedtime ***
- Unison Capsules – one at bedtime**

Vitamins

- Vitamin Code Raw B Complex by Garden of Life; contains probiotics and enzymes to help digestion – one a day in the morning ****
- Vitamin B12 – one tab a day ****
- Biotin, 30 mg capsules – one a day to help hair growth and nails ****
- Multivitamin and minerals by Life Extension ****

Probiotics

- Probiotics by Garden of Life Dr. Formulated 50 Billion – one capsule a day****

Probiotics are good bacteria in the gut that help to improve your immune system; reduce gas; help the digestive system; help absorb nutrients, vitamins, and minerals; and help with production of enzymes and other nutrients.

Fish oil / omega-3

You should take this essential fatty acid every day for optimal health.

- Fish Oil Ultra High Potency EPA/DHA 1,500 mg smoothie by Barlean's – one teaspoon in orange juice every morning, comes in various flavors (lime, passion pineapple, mango, and peach) ****

- Fish Oil with Vitamin D EPA/DHA 720 mg smoothie by Barlean's, mango peach ****
- Fish Oil Total Omega 3-6-9 365 mg smoothie by Barlean's, orange cream ***
- Flax Oil Vegan Formula Smoothie LNA 2,968 mg, mango or strawberry banana ****
- Krill oil soft gels 500 mg by Nature's Way ****

Rejuvenation supplements for stem cells

These supplements and antioxidants will help stem cell activity to keep your stem cells healthy and ready to fight for you and reverse aging.

- To boost AMPK, Curcumin by CuraMed; BCM 95 soft gels – twice a day ****
- AMPK activator by Life Extension, signals cells to use fat – one tablet a day ****
- Green tea, matcha, *Gynostemma*, hesperidin.
- To boost cellular NAD+, Nicotinamide riboside by Life Extension – 250 mg capsules twice a day ****
- To boost SIRT, Resveratrol by Life Extension – 100–250 caps mg a day ****

Herbs and Supplement Combinations, Creams, Gels, and other Medicines Classified by Problems or Diseases

Use these products alone or in combination for better results. I make these recommendations based on my experience. There are many botanicals and combinations and it is very difficult to say which are the best for different problems. The most effective ones are listed here. Check with your physician for interactions or side effects with other medicines you may be taking. These are guides and not a substitution for medical treatment with more effective medications. Herbs are popular in European countries and prescribed by doctors. Chinese and Indian medicine are very rich in herbal medicines.

Acne

Salicylic acid creams and cleansers, benzoyl peroxide creams, retinoid creams and gels, antibiotic creams and gels, Accutane, yeast (*Saccharomyces cerevisiae*), chromium picolinate

Anemia

Iron; zinc; iodized salt; vitamins A, B2, B6, B9 (folic acid), B12, and C

Anxiety, stress, depression, and memory

Echinacea angustifolia root extract tablets, B complex vitamin, omega-3, choline, magnesium, SAM-e, Gotu kola, ashwagandha, GABA, valerian root, rosemary caps and teas, holy basil, Adrenal Health by Gaia that contains *Rhodiola* and holy basil, kava, *Bacopa*, ginkgo, hops, lemon balm

Alzheimer's

Bacopa, ginkgo, lemon balm, turmeric, vitamin B1(benfotiamine)

Arthritis

Omega-3, glucosamine with chondroitin, SAM-e, CoQ10, B complex vitamins, calcium, magnesium, selenium, zinc, turmeric (curcumin), vitamin D, willow bark, turmeric, black cohosh, devil's claw, ginger, vitamin E, hyaluronic acid injections

Blood flow

L-arginine, nitric oxide, citrulline, watermelon

Bad cholesterol and high lipids

Niacin, statins (medication), omega-3, beta-glucagon, psyllium (Metamucil), holy basil, dark chocolate, bilberries, garlic, yeast flakes

Bruising, edema, and venous insufficiency

Grape seed

Constipation

Magnesium citrate, probiotics, psyllium (Metamucil), Smooth Move Tea

Coughs, colds

Many herbal teas are helpful, including, echinacea, peppermint, ginger, and licorice with lemon tea (helps with congestion); zinc tablets and zinc lozenges; mix black elderberry, ginger tea, and honey for cough and congestion; vitamin C (500 mg)

Diabetes

Aloe, cinnamon, alpha lipoic acid, Siberian ginseng, stevia, psyllium, ashwagandha, holy basil, chromium picolinate, berberine 500 mg caps, Gymnema extract, AMPK tablets

Diarrhea

Fluids with electrolytes (sodium, potassium, and chloride); probiotics; bilberries caps and teas; blueberries; garlic

Diuretic

Hibiscus, parsley caps and teas

Endothelial health and plaque formation

Vitamin K2 and K7

Eye health

Vitamin A, B complex vitamin, zinc, bilberries, omega-3, biotin

Fatigue

Rhodiola, rosemary, valerian, ashwagandha, Asian ginseng, B complex vitamin, B12, CoQ10, GABA, Gotu kola, Adrenal Health by Gaia (with *Rhodiola* and holy basil)

Fibromyalgia

Salt with iodine, melatonin, SAM-e, vitamin D, magnesium, Gotu kola, melatonin, lemon balm, choline, hops, valerian root extract

Hypertension

- Diuretic herbs that lower blood pressure – hibiscus, parsley, grapes, grape seeds
- Vasodilators that lower blood pressure – L-arginine, citrulline, nitric oxide
- Antianxiety supplements that help to lower blood pressure – those above, fish oil, CoQ10, hawthorn, beets

Headaches and migraines

Feverfew and butterbur, magnesium

Heartburn, gastritis

Chamomile, licorice, peppermint, calcium bicarbonate, carbonate soda, garlic for *H. Pylori*, melatonin

Hot flashes during menopause

Multivitamin with minerals, B12, vitamins D and K, calcium, magnesium, choline, melatonin, zinc, omega-3, GABA, *Bacopa*, Gotu kola

Insomnia, sleeping

Lemon balm; hops; passionflower; valerian in drops and teas; skullcap; ashwagandha; Gotu kola; melatonin drops and sublingual tablets of 1 to 3 mg one hour before bedtime; magnesium, 400 mg caps; chamomile or valerian teas with a pinch of skullcap, one or two bags at night forty-five minutes before bedtime

Inflammation, joint pain

Turmeric (curcumin), ginger, cinnamon, hops, ashwagandha, glucosamine, omega-3, vitamin D, SAM-e

Menstrual cramps, menopausal symptoms

Black cohosh teas and capsules, black haw, dong quai, fennel, chamomile, hops, vitamin B6, calcium, magnesium, choline, omega-3, selenium, zinc, *Bacopa*, GABA, resveratrol, Gotu kola, *Rhodiola*

Muscle cramps and aches

Black haw; peppermint; magnesium; CoQ10; SAM-e; vitamins B1, D, and E

Neuropathy and nerve pain

B complex vitamins, CoQ10, L-arginine

Prostate problems

Zinc, vitamin D, saw palmetto

Stress

Gotu kola; *Rhodiola*; ashwagandha; Adrenal Health from Gaia Herbs; *Bacopa*; GABA, quick acting

Swelling and bruising

Arnica

APPENDIX C
Hair and Skin Care for a Younger Look

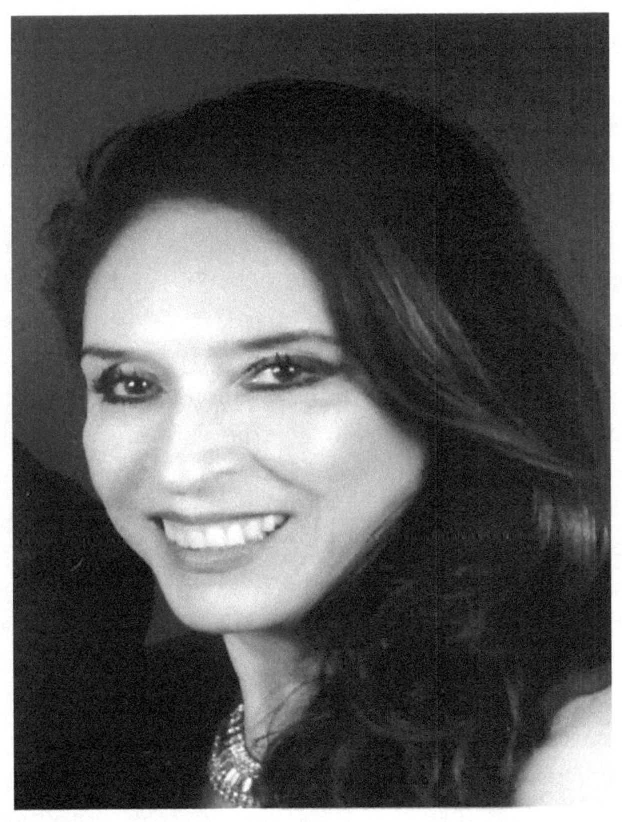

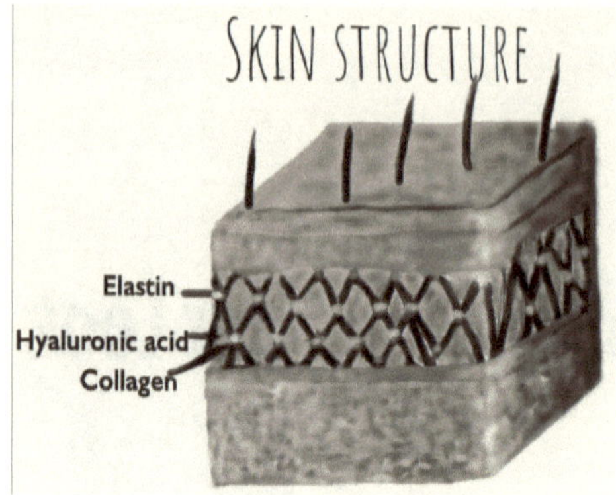

How Wrinkles Develop

Under the surface of the skin, a second layer called the dermis is where the skin makes the scaffolds that prevent wrinkles. These scaffolds are made of collagen and elastin. If one element is lacking, the scaffold becomes weak or breaks, causing wrinkles.

Avoid the sun and cigarette smoking. Polyphenols found in green tea and green veggies slow down the MMP enzymes, which reduce collagen as you age.

Keep your skin healthy to look younger

To slow down or stop the signs of aging, keep your skin healthy. It is important to use a good moisturizer and sunscreen every day. UV rays from too much sun exposure cause over 80 percent of skin damage that makes you look older. To prevent this damage, use sunscreen with an SPF (sun protection factor) of 30 or higher. Sunscreen must protect against UVA and UVB radiation. Oils do not offer good protection. In fact, oils allow deeper penetration of UV rays. The best UVB absorbers contain homosalate, octisalate, octocrylene, and avobenzone. Water-resistant sunscreens contain silicones (dimethicone) or a polymer (sodium polyacrylate) to give more staying power when you are in the water or sweating a great deal. Sunscreens also contain zinc oxide and titanium dioxide. Some contain Mexoryl SX, recently approved by the FDA.

Small cells called fibroblasts make collagen. The matrix metalloproteinases (MMPs) are part of the larger family of metalloproteinase enzymes that play an important part in wound healing. These enzymes break down proteins under the skin and affect healing (Gibson Wounds International 2009).

MMP enzymes break down collagen, but too much activity of these enzymes decreases collagen, resulting in wrinkles and skin healing. Retinoids from vitamin A usually bind with receptors in the fibroblasts, helping to turn off the MMP enzymes. If you are developing wrinkles, use a retinoid cream every night with a moisturizer. Peptides, which are small chains of amino acids, help to increase the production of collagen. Creams with peptides are useful to prevent wrinkles. In one study reported in the *New England Journal of Medicine*, sun-damaged skin treated for about a year with tretinoin (the active ingredient of Retin A) had an 80 percent increase in collagen compared to a 14 percent decrease treated with a placebo cream. Many studies found that the use of a .02 percent cream over 24 weeks significantly improved fine wrinkles.

Vitamin C creams make the skin smooth due to the antioxidants effects. Vitamin C plays an important role in collagen production. Vitamin E is also helpful, since it provides essential oils that moisturize the skin. CoQ10 and idebenone are powerful antioxidants in topical skin products, which are better than vitamin C and E when used to decrease wrinkles.

When the wrinkles are deep, Botox is better and very effective. For larger areas and folds, injections of hyaluronic acid as fillers help to hide deep folds for twelve months. Restylane-L and Juvederm are some of these products. Restylane seems to last longer than Juvederm to remove wrinkles. A product called Sculptra may last up to five years.

For sagging skin, ultrasound radio frequency and light energy devices help to increase collagens that make the skin taut. It works better in cases of mild to moderate skin laxity.

For daily use, I recommend creams, serum, and gels with hyaluronic acid. Apply this cream day and night for better results. Use it with a moisturizing cream and a sunscreen. Green tea is rich in antioxidants like polyphenols and flavonoids, which help to prevent skin damage and wrinkles.

The caffeine in coffee helps to reduce inflammation and puffy eyes. Dab some coffee in a tissue and apply it to the lower eyelids to relieve puffiness, particularly after a trip or reduced sleep. I also recommend a hyaluronic acid cream, serum, or gel under the eyelids to remove puffiness and wrinkles. It works fast, and the effect may last a few hours. I personally apply hyaluronic acid serum to my face and let it dry before using a moisturizer at night and in the morning. At night, I also use a 2.5 percent retinol serum around the eyes.

Dark spots

The sun activates your melanocytes to make them produce a dark pigment that travels to the surface of your skin. The more exposure to the sun, the greater the activity of melanocytes and the production of pigment. To stop the activity of the melanocytes, avoid sun exposure and use a cream containing hydroquinone, which inhibits the enzyme tyrosinase responsible for the production of the pigment. Apply a hydroquinone cream for day and night use to decrease the activity of the melanocytes. To prevent dark spots and skin damage, you should use a sunscreen with an SPF of 30. A .025 percent retinol cream applied every night helps to remove dark spots and remove small wrinkles. Check the content of the sunscreen to be sure it has the recommendations above for better protection. Also avoid sunburns and tanning salons to prevent dark spots.

Hair growth and baldness

Men with higher levels of dihydrotestosterone (DHT) have increased levels of hair loss. Too much of this hormone can shrink hair follicles to the point where no new hair can grow. Men may notice baldness of the crown of the head as the first sign of baldness. Rogaine stimulates hair growth in men by inhibiting the activity of DHT. Rogaine works better with early signs of baldness. Once baldness is total, it does not work.

Two preparations (2 percent and 5 percent) rubbed into the hair work about the same. However, recent studies found that, after a year of daily use, 5 percent Rogaine works better than the 2 percent preparation. Some drugs used to treat the enlargement of the prostate help to decrease baldness, but they have some side effects. Propecia and Avodart help to inhibit DHT. *Women should not use these drugs.*

Spot baldness, alopecia areata or patchy hair loss, may affect some women. When a woman is losing hair, she may be under a great deal of stress. Reducing stress helps to improve this condition. Pulling the hair to create a ponytail too tightly may cause hair loss. Low thyroid may be associated with hair loss. Steroid creams may help to improve hair loss.

Garlic gels twice a day, combined with a steroid cream, were helpful in men treated in a placebo-controlled study in Iran. Onion juice has been found to stimulate hair growth. Some hair shampoos, conditioners, and serums also promote hair growth. Saw palmetto is a DHT inhibitor. I recommend saw palmetto extract, which you can find in health stores. Use five drops of the extract in 10 ml of water and apply it to the hair after using a shampoo and conditioner to thicken the hair. You can use a serum to thicken the hair after the application. Supplementation with zinc and biotin is recommended. Shampoos and conditioners containing biotin are helpful to keep hair stronger and prevent hair loss.

Smoothies

Vegetable-fruit smoothies

Green Delight for the Family

Ingredients
1/2 cup kale
1/2 cup spinach
1 cup slide apples
1/2 banana
1/2 cup pineapple chunks
2 cups of water
2 cups of apple juice (Old Orchard healthy balance)

Directions
Mix in a blender on high for one minute. Add more water to thin.

Notes

Old Orchard brand offers a reduced sugar juice (4 g) to cut calories.

- Substitute bananas for 1 cup of frozen strawberries or blueberries to enjoy different flavors.

- These smoothies are a way to add vegetables to children's diets. Schools should provide these smoothies instead of sodas or juices rich in sugars, since they provide a healthier blend of vegetables and fruits, which are refreshing and palatable.
- This smoothie has fiber to lower the carbs in the fruits. Kale and spinach are rich in protein, calcium, and vitamin K, with high nutritional value. See tables 1 and 2, in chapter 2 on diet.
- For more fiber, add two teaspoons of Metamucil or brewer's yeast flakes to the mix and blend. Brewer's yeast is rich in amino acids and minerals and provides additional fiber.

Dr. P's recommendation to make healthy smoothies

This is a basic veggie-fruit smoothie. You can make high protein shakes from this basic smoothie. The shakes are recommended as a meal for children, very active young adults, muscle builders, patients recovering from illness or injuries, and active athletic people suffering from inflammation. The smoothie contains veggies, bromelian from pineapple, which is an anti-inflammatory.

To prepare the high protein veggie shake, add 1 to 2 cups of light almond or unsweetened coconut milk and 1 to 2 scoops of superfood protein from Ground-Based Nutrition. This protein is made from plants and contains no diary or soy. It also contains fiber and veggies, is gluten free, and has no sugar.

As an alternative, you can use 2 percent milk, unsweetened soy milk, or almond milk that contains many amino acids required for a balanced diet. I also recommend brewer's yeast, available as flakes, since the flakes provide most essential amino acids and minerals like chromium that helps to improve insulin sensitivity, increase HDL, and lower triglycerides. Chromium helps to improve acne, very common in adolescents.

Shakes can be taken twice a day. They can be used for weight control since the smoothies are low in carbohydrates and fats, contain fiber, and have all the amino acids, vitamins, and minerals for normal function. If you want to lose weight, keep carbs below 15 grams per serving. Always be aware of the glycemic index of many fruits.

Drinks and low-carb smoothies

Morning Essentials

Ingredients
1/2 cup fresh squeezed orange juice
1 teaspoon omega-3 fish oil or flaxseed oil (Barlean brand)

Directions
Mix in a glass to start your day with the essentials.

Notes

- This is a great drink to stay healthy and keep your body strong, reduce inflammation, help your body to repair cell membranes and cartilage, and maintain a healthy heart. I recommend 50 percent reduced sugar orange juice, squeezed oranges, or diet apple juice. Fish oil and flaxseed oil are available in different flavors and are packed with omega-3. We prefer the Barlean brand because it offers many flavors and reduced calories.
- Vitamin C and omega-3 are two essential vital nutrients. My wife and I drink this smoothie every morning. You can add yeast flakes to add more amino acids and minerals like chromium, magnesium, calcium, and selenium. You can find the Barlean brand in vitamin and health food stores.

Libido-Muscle Power Smoothie

Ingredients
1/2 watermelon
1 tablespoon shelled sunflower seeds
2 teaspoons L-arginine powder
1/2 cup ice
2 cups water

Directions
Blend at high speed for one minute. Makes 4 cups of smoothie.

Notes

- Watermelon is rich in citrulline and L-arginine. Both amino acids help to raise nitric oxide, a vasodilator, which in turns improves libido, lowers blood pressure, and improves circulation.
- Be careful if you use nitrates for angina or have low blood pressure.

Citrus Strawberry Smoothie

Ingredients
1 cup squeezed orange juice
1 cup squeezed red grapefruit juice
1 cup frozen strawberries
1/3 cup shelled sunflower seeds
1 tablespoon flaxseed oil (available in many flavors)
I cup sugar-free yogurt
1 cup water

Directions
– Mix the ingredients in a blender and blend for 45 seconds at high speed.
– Garnish with a strawberry if desired. Add stevia to your taste if desired.
This preparation yields 4 cups. Using more water and more sesame seeds for fiber helps to lower the carbs intake.

Notes

This smoothie is rich in vitamins A, B, B6, and E; magnesium, manganese, selenium, zinc, and copper; and omega-3 and cysteine. Plus, it has lots of antioxidants. It's great to strengthen your immune system.

Mango Sensational Smoothie

Ingredients
2 cups mango pulp
2 cups water
2 tablespoons sesame seeds
1 cup sugar-free yogurt

1 tablespoon stevia

1 cup ice

Directions

Mix ingredients in the blender and blend for 45 seconds at high speed.

Notes

- Sesame seeds provide fiber to decrease the carbs in a mango.
- You can buy fresh mangos to get the pulp or buy the pulp ready for use.

***

Goya Foods in the Mexican section offers many frozen fruits for juices ready to blend. Many supermarkets offer fruits and veggies already in a packet ready to blend. You can make your own in a plastic bag.

Try a different smoothie for each day of the week.

Mixing fruits and vegetables can provide both elements of a low-carb diet, as well as fiber. As a rule, my wife and I are 60 to 70 percent vegetarians. Beside smoothies, we add fish, poultry, and eggs to our diets for a more balanced diet. Fiber is important to lower the carb load.

I recommend that you check tables 1 and 2 in chapter 2 on diet for the content of antioxidants and carbs for many fruits. If you are on a diet, keep carbs below 15 g when making smoothies. If you want to be stricter, your total amount of carbs per day should not exceed more than 30 g.

On the contrary, if you are recovering from an illness or need to gain weight, you can be more liberal with your carbs, unless you are diabetic. Add plant powder to the smoothies to gain weight or muscle mass. If you exercise or want to develop muscle mass, increase the amount of protein. I recommend plant protein products since they contain most of the amino acids and minerals required in a well-balanced diet. I also recommend brewer's yeast in the form of yeast flakes or powder made from *Saccharomyces cerevisiae* for more amino acids and minerals like chromium and selenium. My wife and I prefer the yeast flakes from KAL, which you can find in vitamin and health food stores.

APPENDIX E
Healthy Desserts

Coconut Blueberry Yogurt

Ingredients
1/2 cup Chobani Greek yogurt
1/2 cup fresh blueberries

Directions
This is an easy dessert to prepare. Use 1/2 cup of coconut nonfat Chobani Greek yogurt and a half cup of fresh blueberries. You can add stevia for a sweet flavor.

Notes
This dessert is rich in antioxidants and probiotics. To add fiber, add a tablespoon of yeast flakes or powder.

Walnuts and Blueberry Cottage Cheese

Ingredients
1/2 cup low-fat cottage cheese
1/2 cup walnuts
1/2 cup fresh blueberries

Directions
In a half cup of low-fat cottage cheese, add a half cup of walnuts and a half cup of blueberries.

Notes

This dessert is rich in antioxidants, calcium, minerals, and proteins. Add stevia for a sweet flavor.

Super Omega-3 Tofu Agave Dessert

Ingredients
1-inch thick slice of hard tofu
1 tablespoon flax-chia blend
1 teaspoon agave

Directions
 – Cut a thick slice of hard tofu in small squares.
 – Sprinkle a tablespoon of flax-chia blend from Garden of Life.
 – Add a teaspoon of agave, and mix.

Notes

Agave has a very low glycemic index and is better than many artificial sweeteners and sugar. The flax-chia blend contains 5 g of fiber, omega-3, antioxidants, calcium, iron, magnesium, and other healthy minerals and is found in vitamin and health food stores.

Brewer's Yeast Flakes Yogurt

Ingredients
1/2 cup light yogurt
1 tablespoon yeast flakes

Directions
Serve a half cup of flavored or nonflavored low-fat yogurt that contains probiotics, add a table spoon of yeast flakes from KAL. Add Stevia powder for additional sweetness and mix.

Brewer's yeast flakes are made by KAL from *Saccharomyces cerevisiae* and are rich in essential amino acids, B vitamins, minerals, and fiber.

You can find this brand of yeast flakes in vitamin and supplement stores.

Coconut-Chia Delight

Ingredients
2 cups coconut milk
1/2 cup chia seeds
1 tablespoon agave syrup
1 teaspoon vanilla extract

Directions
- Mix the ingredients in a jar, cover tightly, and shake the mix.
- Place the jar in the refrigerator for at least 30 minutes or leave overnight for 12 hours.
- Serve with blueberries or fruit and/or Stevia or more agave for sweetness (optional).

Notes

Coconut-Chia Delight can be used for breakfast as well.

A Healthy Salad

Nice Sleep Salad

Prepare a salad with spinach, kale, avocado, almonds, walnuts, pineapple, and orange chunks. Add balsamic vinaigrette and olive oil. For more protein, add salmon or chicken.

This salad contains sufficient magnesium, calcium and L-tryptophan, the main amino acid and precursor of serotonin and melatonin. It helps to increase levels of melatonin during the night and restore your normal circadian rhythm at night.

Avoid refined sugars and too many carbs at night, since they raise the levels of insulin, which interferes with your sleep.

Resources

Screening and blood testing

Quest and Lab Corp are national laboratories used by most doctors nationwide for almost any kind of lab testing.

Life Extension
Website: www.lifeextension.com

Private MD Labs
Website: www.privatemdlabs.com

Telomere testing

Telomere diagnostic
Website: teloyears.com
Offers telomere and ancestry DNA testing; telomere testing less than $100

DNA testing

Ancestry
Website: ancestry.com
Offers DNA testing

Genetic testing

23andme
23andme.com

Mayo Clinic
Website: mayoclinic.org
Offers diagnostic and genetic testing for specific diseases or conditions

REFERENCES

Books and general articles of interest researched

American Diabetes Association. n.d. "Glycemic Index and Diabetes." www. diabetes.org/food-and-fitness/food/what-can-i-eat/understanding-carbohydrates/glycemic-index-and-diabetes.html?loc=ff-slabnav. Accessed May 18, 2016.

Bodkin, Henry. 2018 "Atkins Diet May Cause Heart Failure." *The Telegraph,* May 29, 2018. https://www.telegraph.co.uk/science/2018/05/29/atkins-diet-may-cause-heart-failure-major-new-protein-study/.

Bergouignan, Audrey. 2016. "Effect of Frequent Interruptions of Prolonged Sitting on Self-Perceived Levels of Energy, Mood, Food Cravings and Cognitive Function." *International Journal of Behavioral Nutrition and Physical Activity,* Nov. 3, 2016. www.ijbnpa.biomedcentral.com/articles/10.1186/s12966-016-0437-z.

Blackburn, Elizabeth, PhD, and Elissa Epel, PhD. 2016. *The Telomere Effect.* New York: Grand Central Publishing.

Braverman, Eric R., MD. 2011. *Younger Brain, Sharper Mind.* New York: Rodale, Inc.

Brody, Jane E. 2016. "The Fight Against Obesity Begins Early." *New York Times,* July 5, 2016, D5.

Chopra Deepak, MD, and David Simon. 2001. *Grow Younger, Live Longer.* New York: Three Rivers Press.

Crowley, Chris, and H. Lodge, MD. 2007. *Younger Next Year.* New York: Workman Publishing.

Downey, Andrea. 2017. "Eating Curry Is Good for You!" www.thesun. co.uk/living/4092612/eating-curry-is-good-for-you-turmeric-helped-cancer-patient-57-beat-myeloma-after-five-years-of-treatment/. *The Sun*. Accessed July 25, 2017.

Dye, Lee. 2012. "Living Longer: Increasing Lifespan May Be in Our Control." ABC News, August 29, 2012. www.abcnews.go.com/Technology/ humans-live-forever-longevity-research-suggests-longer-life/ story?id=17100148.

Esmonde-White, Miranda. 2014. *Aging Backwards*. New York: Harper Collins.

Esselstyn, Caldwell B., Jr., MD. 2008. *Prevent and Reverse Heart Disease*. New York: Penguin Group, 64–71.

Fox News. 2017. "No Fruit Juice for Kids under 1, Doctors Say." Fox News Health, May 22, 2017. www.foxnews.com/health/2017/05/22/no-fruit-juice-for-kids-under-1-doctors-say.html.

Genome.gov https://www.genome.gov/19016938/faq-about-genetics-disease -prevention-and-treatment/

Gibson, D., B. Cullen, R. Legerstee, K. G. Harding, and G. Schultz. 2009. "MMPs Made Easy." *Wounds International* 1, no. 1. Available from http:// www.woundsinternational.com.

Guay, André, and Susan Davis. 2002. "Testosterone Insufficiency Fact or Fiction?" *World Journal of Urology*. http://www.bumc.bu.edu/sexualmedicine/ publications/testosterone-insufficiency-in-women-fact-or-fiction/.

Guerrero, G. P., M. M. Zago, N. O. Sawada, and M. H. Pinto. 2011. "Relationship between Spirituality and Cancer: Patient's Perspective." *Rev Bras Enferm* 64, no. 1: 53–59.

Gundry, Steven R., MD. 2017. *The Plant Paradox*. New York: Harper Collins Publishers.

Haden, S. T., J. Glowacki, S. Hurwitz, C. Rosen, and M. S. LeBoff. 2000. "Effects of Age on Serum Dehydroepiandrosterone Sulfate, IGF-I, and IL-6 levels in Women." *Calcif Tissue Int* 66, no. 6 (June): 414–18.

Head, K. A. 1998. "Estriol: Safety and Efficacy." *Altern Med Rev* 3, no. 2 (April): 101–13.

Heid Markham, O'Connor Siobhan, editor. 2015. _Secrets of Living Longer_. Time Inc. Books, 21–25.

Horner, Christine, MD. 2016. *Radiant Health Ageless Beauty*. San Diego: Elgea Publishing.

Hotze Steve, MD. 2103. *Hormones, Health, and Happiness*. Charleston, SC: Advantage Media Group.

Hyman, Mark, M.D. 2016. *Eat Fat, Get Thin.* New York: Little Brown and Company.Jenkins, J. A. 2016. *Disrupt Aging.* First Edition. New York: Public Affairs.

Ironson, G., G. F. Solomon, E. G. Balbin, et al. 2002. The Ironson-Woods Spirituality/Religiousness Index Is Associated with Long Survival, Health Behaviors, Less Distress, and Low Cortisol in People with HIV/AIDS." *Ann Behav Med* 24, no. 1: 34–48.

Kalamian Miriam, EdM, MS, CNS. 2017. *Keto for Cancer.* Chelsea Green Publishing.

Kolata, Gina. 2016. "Diabetes and Your Diet: The Low-Carb Debate." *New York Times*, September 16, 2016. www.nytimes.com/2016/09/16/health/type-2-diabetes-low-carb-diet.html Accessed September 9, 2016.

Kramer, Leslie. 2017. "One Third of Americans Are Headed for Diabetes, and They Don't Even Know It." CNBC.com, August 17, 2017. www.medicalxpress.com/news/2016-07-fruit-vegetables-substantially-happiness.html.

Kummer, Sebastian, MD, Derik Hermsen, MD, and Felix Distelmaier, MD. 2016. "Biotin Treatment Mimicking Grave's Disease." Massachusetts Medical Society, August 18, 2016. www.nejm.org/doi/full/10.1056/NEJMc1602096?query=endocrinology

Larimore, W. L., M. Parker, and M. Crowther. 2002. "Should Clinicians Incorporate Positive Spirituality into their Practices? What Does the Evidence Say?" *Ann Behav Med* 24, no. 1: 69–73.

Lawler-Row, K. A., and J. Elliott. 2009. "The Role of Religious Activity and Spirituality in the Health and Well-Being of Older Adults." *J Health Psychol* 14, no. 1: 43–52.

Longo, Valter, PhD. 2018. *The Longevity Diet.* New York: Penguin & Random House LLC, 214–16.

LowDog, Tieraona, MD. 2016. *Fortify Your Life.* Washington, DC: National Geographic Society.

Mayo Clinic. 2018. Hormone Therapy: Is It Right for You? https://www.mayoclinic.org/diseases-conditions/menopause/in-depth/hormone-therapy/ART-20046372.

McCall, Becky. 2017. "Vitamin D Supplements May Raise Sex Hormone Levels in Men." *Medscape*, June 01, 2017. European Congress of Endocrinology (ECE) (2017).

Mercola, Joseph. 2017. *Fat for Fuel.* Carlsbad, CA: Hay House Inc.

Meyer, Joyce. 2015. *The Mind Connection.* New York: Faith Words Hachette Book Group.

Mizushima N. 2007 "Autophagy: Process and Function." *Gen Dev.* 21, no 22: 2861–73.

McVay, M. R. 2002. "Medicine and Spirituality: A Simple Path to Restore Compassion in Medicine." *SDJ Med 55*, no. 11: 487–91.

Morales, A. J., J. J. Nolan, J.C. Nelson, and S. S. Yen. 1994. "Effects of Replacement Dose of Dehydroepiandrosterone in Men and Women of Advancing Age." *J Clin Endocrinol Metab* 78, no. 6 (June): 1360–67.

Murphy Helen, editor. 2018. "Is Your Nitric Oxide Supplement Effective?" www. consumereview.org/nitric-oxide/nitric-oxide-supplement-effective/.

Murray, Michael, ND. 2017. *The Magic of Food.* New York: Atria Books, Simon &Schuster Inc.

National Institutes of Health (NIH) Office of Dietary Supplements. 2018. "Vitamin E: Fact Sheet for Health Professionals." https://ods.od.nih.gov/ factsheets/VitaminE-HealthProfessional/.

Nelson, C. J., B. J. Rosenfeld, W. Breitbart, and M. Galietta. 2002. "Spirituality, Religion, and Depression in the Terminally Ill." *Psychosomatics* 43, no. 3: 213–20.

Noto H., A. Goto, T. Tsujimoto, and M. Noda. 2013. "Low-Carbohydrate Diets and All-Cause Mortality: A Systematic Review and Meta-Analysis of Observational Studies." *PLoS ONE* 8, no. 1: e55030. https://doi. org/10.1371/journal.pone.0055030.

Park, Alice and Siobhan-Marie O'Connor. 2015. *How to Live to Be 100: Secrets of Living Longer.* Time Inc. Books.

Reader's Digest Best Health. n.d. "40 Foods High in Antioxidants." Originally "Anti-Oxidant-Rich Fare" in *Best Health Magazine* (January/February 2009). Accessed March 6, 2018. www.besthealthmag.ca/best-eats/ nutrition/40-foods-high-in-antioxidants/.

Reivich, Karen, and Andrew Shatte. 2002. *The Resilience Factor.* NJ: Bright & Happy Books, LLC.

Renner, Ben. 2017. "Artificial Sweeteners Stimulate Fat Growth, Harmful to Metabolism, Study Finds." December 13, 2017. www.studyfinds.org/ sweeteners-fat-growth-obesity/.

Reynolds, Gretchen. 2017. "Work. Walk 5 Minutes. Work." *New York Times,* January 3, 2017, D4. www.nytimes.com/2016/12/28/well/move/work-walk-5-minutes-work.html?_r=0.

Romanoski, Anya. 2018. "Ketogenic Diet: Which patients benefit?" *Medscape.* https://www.medscape.com/viewarticle/894041_4. Accessed March 24, 2018.

Salas-Salvadó, Jordi et al. 2016. "Protective Effects of the Mediterranean Diet on Type 2 Diabetes and Metabolic Syndrome." *The Journal of Nutrition* 146, no. 4: 920S–927S. *PMC.* Web. March 5, 2018.

Sesink, Aloys L. A., Denise S. M. L. Termont, Jan H. Kleibeuker and Roelof Van der Meer. 1999. "Red Meat and Colon Cancer." *Cancer Research* (November). http://cancerres.aacrjournals.org/content/59/22/5704.

Sheldrick, Giles. 2016. "Eat Nuts to Live Longer." Accessed December 6, 2016. www.express.co.uk/life-style/health/739777/Eat-nuts-live-longer-doctors-prescribe-fight-killer-diseases-heart-disease-cancer-obesity.

Sleiman, Dana, Marwa R. Al-Badri, and Sami T. Azar. 2015. "Effect of Mediterranean Diet in Diabetes Control and Cardiovascular Risk Modification: A Systematic Review." *Frontiers in Public Health* 3: 69. *PMC.* Web. March 5, 2018.

"Spirituality." www.umm.edu/health/medical/altmed/treatment/spirituality. February 1, 2018.

Steingold, Daniel. 2017. "Study: Artificial Sweeteners Linked to Weight Gain, Other Health Problems." July 17, 2017. www.studyfinds.org/artificial-sweeteners-weight-gain-heart/.

Taubes, Gary. 2016. *The Case Against Sugar.* New York: Alfred A Knopf Publisher, a division of Penguin Random House, LLC., 258–262.

Tay, J., Luscombe-Marsh, ND, C. H. Thompson, M. Noakes, J. D. Buckley, G. A. Wittert, W. S. Yancy Jr., and G. D. Brinkworth, G.D. 2015 "Comparison of Low- and High-Carbohydrate Diets for Type 2 Diabetes Management: A Randomized Trial." *The American Journal of Clinical Nutrition* 102, 780–90. http://dx.doi.org/10.3945/ajcn.115.112581.

Weber, Robert, PhD, and Carol Orsborn, PhD. 2015. *The Spirituality of Age.* Rochester, VT: Park Street Press.

Young, Anthony, MD. 2016. *The Age Fix.* New York: Grand Central Life & Style.

INDEX